Secrets of an
Alkaline Body

Secrets of an Alkaline Body

*The New
Science of
Colloidal
Biology*

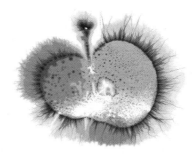

ANNIE PADDEN JUBB AND DAVID JUBB, PH.D.

North Atlantic Books
Berkeley, California

Published by
North Atlantic Books
P.O. Box 12327
Berkeley, California 94712

Cover and book design by Jan Camp
Kirlean photographs by Chris Wodtke

Printed in the United States of America

Secrets of an Alkaline Body is sponsored by the Society for the Study of Native Arts and Sciences, a nonprofit educational corporation whose goals are to develop an educational and crosscultural perspective linking various scientific, social, and artistic fields; to nurture a holistic view of arts, sciences, humanities, and healing; and to publish and distribute literature on the relationship of mind, body, and nature.

North Atlantic Books' publications are available through most bookstores. For further information, call 800-733-3000 or visit our website at www.northatlanticbooks.com.

ISBN-13: 978-1-55643-481-5

Library of Congress Cataloging-in-Publication Data

Jubb, Annie Padden.
Secrets of an alkaline body : the new science of colloidal biology /
    by Annie Padden Jubb & David Jubb.
        p. cm.
    ISBN 1-55643-481-2 (pbk.)
    1. Cancer—Etiology—Popular works. 2. Alkalosis—Complications—Popular works. 3. Colloids—Physiological effect—Popular works. 4. Infection—Complications—Popular works. 5. Metabolic detoxification—Popular works.
    [DNLM: 1. Neoplasms—diet therapy. 2. Colloids—metabolism. 3. Dietary Supplements. 4. Minerals—metabolism. 5. Neoplasms—blood. 6. Nutrition. QZ 266 J91s 2003] I. Jubb, David. II. Title.
    RC268.48.J83 2003
    616.99'4071—dc22

                                                                    2003019722
                                                                        CIP
        5 6 7 8 9 10 11 DATA 12 11 10 09 08

Acknowledgments

To all healers and researchers who dedicate their lives to the health and forwarded consciousness of humankind.

And most especially in loving memory of William R. Fair, M.D.

IMPORTANT NOTE

This material is educational advice to help you live a full healthy life. Remember, a health professional is only a consultant. You have the first and last word for your health.

A health and cleansing program should make sense to you before adopting it and only you can decide if something is right for you. The use of good common sense and accountability for one's own health is assumed here.

To contact the authors send correspondence to: Jubbs Longevity, Inc. 508 East 12th Street, New York City, NY 10009-3891. Phone 212.353.5000 and 212.353.5015.

LIFEFOOD RECIPES

All recipes referenced in this book, can be found in *LifeFood Recipe Book: Living on LifeFood*, North Atlantic Books, 2003

Table of Contents

Contents

Contents

Introduction

Microscopes offer a fascinating look inward, a window into well-ordered worlds—strange and surreal, yet governed by natural cosmic law. There is great order in nature.

Where the laws of nature have been overlooked we find disease (dis-ease: a disruption to ease). There is only one disease: toxicity and enervation, a lack of nerve force. When people indulge in too many toxic chemicals, drugs, denatured foods, pollution, and stress and don't allow for or forget to get enough LifeFood Nutrition, fresh air and sunshine, pure water, relaxation, exercise, and passion, they are overlooking natural law and won't feel well.

LifeFood Nutrition is advocated in this book. It is good for you and the Earth because it is completely in harmony with natural law. Life-Food is fresh, delicious, organically grown food that is good for the land, promoting shade-bearing vegetation that rejuvenates soil and contributes to purifying lakes, rivers, and oceans. LifeFood offers the highest quality nutrition on Earth because it is so natural. You really can't improve upon nature. I chuckle sometimes when people or institutions hold themselves above nature. We are all bound by the laws of nature because the human is nature itself, as everything that grows on Earth is. We occupy these bodies while we are here and leave them behind when we go, for they belong to the Earth.

In our book *LifeFood Recipe Book: Living on Life Force,* David and I outline this way of living and eating and describe in common terms how the LifeFood diet is the ultimate healing program. It includes 200 recipes that are delicious and easy to prepare. We also describe our signature 14-Day LifeFood Nutritional Fast that includes gallbladder and liver flushes—an incredible way to jumpstart any healing program for quick recovery from modern dietary excesses. It will leave you feeling rejuvenated and looking radiant. The LifeFood Nutritional Fast is the ultimate healing and beautification program that entails flooding the body with colloidal nutrients in blended beverages (fresh soups, smoothies, our signature *Electrolyte Lemonade,* nutmilks, sun tea) that are incredibly easy for the body to absorb and assimilate. At the same time this fast liquefies deep-lying toxins (mucous, wax, heavy metal, chemicals, gallstones, fecal mucoid matter) and whisks them away. It encourages plenty of trips to the bathroom (3 to 5 per day) as this material exits the body.

We encourage you to read *LifeFood Recipe Book* because we assume a basic understanding of LifeFood Nutrition here. In this book, we go into detail to describe how mold, fungus, and yeast are the chief undertakers of nature and how to jumpstart a sluggish immune system. We describe herbal formulas that contain complex phytonutrients, designed by nature to clean up the blood and rejuvenate lymph functioning.

The brain and money drain in health research today is astounding. Most research money goes toward drugs and surgery. This approach completely ignores the laws of nature. Natural law states that a boosted immune system restores health. Most of this research money could be going into boosting immunity. The body is a perfect self-correcting mechanism; remove toxins and bring up natural electrical functioning and health returns. Drugs and surgery are wonderful for trauma injuries; however, they will never cure cancer or any other disease. If they could, they would have done so by now. More than thirty years of cancer research and hundreds and hundreds of billions of dollars later, and still no "magic bullet" that cures cancer.

And yet, there are thousands of people who have healed their own cancers and other diseases spontaneously. Nearly everyone in this group reports making sweeping changes in their lives in several areas: diet, exercise, environment, relationships, career, etc. They rooted out the toxic areas of their lives and made changes. Across the board, they were people who decided they had the power within them to heal their condition. They called up a very strong conviction to live.

We are complex creatures ruled by simple natural law. All the money that goes into the "magic bullet" to kill cancer would be silly were it not so tragic. The war on cancer is making the profiteers in the drug industry rich beyond imagine, and humanity is its casualty. There is only one disease: toxicity and enervation, which is a lack of nerve force. If an animal in the wild has cancer, we automatically know that the cause must be that their food, water, and/or environment is polluted. Investigators find the source of the pollution to eliminate it, and the animal recovers. The propaganda about cancer is such that you'd think a person could just be walking innocently down the street one day and suddenly get attacked with cancer. Nonsense. While it's true a person could be poisoned, it is far more common for cancer and all metabolic diseases to form slowly and over a long period of time from a constant pattern of overlooking natural law.

LifeFood Nutrition boosts the immune system, dissolves toxins to debulk the body, and floods the body with highly absorbable colloidal vitamins and minerals. This sets the stage for remission. Modern medicine approaches cancer by flooding the body with known toxins and trying to bring the immune system to within an inch of death before attempting to revive it. Cancer is primarily treated with surgery, and radiation and chemotherapy, which are known toxins. Surgery is an overused procedure of cutting out body parts that are desperately trying to do their job.

Gallbladder removal is one of the most overused surgeries. It is very popular today to remove the gallbladder simply because a person has gallstones. It is the job of the gallbladder, the trashcan for the liver, to accumulate this material until the liver can sufficiently process it so it can be effectively eliminated. Gallstones are caused from a diet of starchy food and a congested liver. The gallbladder and liver flushes we promote are highly efficient in clearing this material away naturally with no medication or surgery, operating in perfect harmony with natural law. Removing healthy gallbladders just because they have gallstones is a shortsighted fix that doesn't begin to address the issues of starchy foods and a congested liver. Add to that the fact that no nutritional recommendations are given to outpatients and you witness a perfect example of the classic modern medical paradigm. The gallbladder is removed and the same gallstone-forming diet continues. This greatly increases the stress load of an already compromised liver and the entire immune system has to work harder. Gallstones will continue to pack into gall ducts where the organ was removed, only to become ever more hardened. Without the gallbladder this material is held longer in the liver and gradually gets dispersed to be stored through the body. A person in this condition will probably live many years less than they might if they practiced body hygiene principles and performed a series of gallbladder flushes.

Overlooking natural law is a "band-aid" approach to medicine. David likes to say that disease is like a sudden cliff at the end of a long road. Every day people come zooming down this road and shoot straight over the cliff, landing with a thud on the canyon floor. Instead of investing in a good fence at the cliff and plenty of warning signs (prevention), modern medicine invests all its resources in ambulances at the canyon floor to cart off the wounded to hospitals for drugs and surgeries.

In the 1800s, there was a running joke about allopathic medicine, "Well, the operation was a great success, but we lost the patient." I've had conversations with top physicians who plainly offer their strategy, "We try to kill the cancer without killing the patient." It's no joke that hospital care is the number three cause of death for Americans. Physicians have taken the Hippocratic oath for thousands of years; it states: "I will prescribe regimen for the good of my patients according to my ability and my judgment and never do harm to anyone." Clearly, trying to "kill the cancer without killing the patient" intends to do harm. It is in violation of natural law to try to kill a part of the body.

The brain drain that funnels into drug research programs commonly ignores cosmic and natural law. These laws must be understood and honored for society to put disease to rest once and for all. When we view a symptom as a teacher, guiding us to discover what we have too much and not enough of, then we solve the mystery, the challenge is over, and we get on with life. When we are healthy, our health is rarely on the mind; when we are unhealthy, we can think of nothing else. LifeFood Nutrition is in perfect harmony with nature; it is loaded with vital electrics and colloidal vitamins and minerals that support and boost the immune system. We are a work in progress, constantly constructing and deconstructing ourselves. LifeFood offers the high quality building materials needed for this constant cycle. It is rich with enzymes, so it costs you nothing to digest, and all of its properties are highly charged and easily utilized.

In this book, David and I focus primarily on the physical aspect of healing, though our backgrounds include a robust investigation into behavior physiology and psychosomatic (body/mind) relations that span two decades. Humans are instinctively social and emotional beings. We live and die for principles and virtues we hold dear, for paradigms we perceive to be real—whether they are or not. This is the nature of humanity, more emotional than rational. Our mind is a collection of belief systems that can be utterly flexible or intensely rigid. The body is the mind's experience of itself. All things thought in the mind have a corresponding physiology in the body.

One important card that is played today in the health game is the manipulation of belief systems through the masterful use of propaganda. The politics of food and medicine are shaped by the heavy hand of propaganda in television and print media. Propaganda utilizes classical hypnoses to engineer belief systems in the mass population to shape a paradigm. There is very little free press left in America today. Television news and newspapers read like office bulletins for multi-national corporations. Popular TV news channels accept large contributions from billion-dollar drug companies to "report" on the "early promising research" for the latest drug for cancer, as if it were breaking news! The value of that particular company's stocks shoots up.

This continues the false pretense that there will, one day, be a drug that cures cancer and that there is no natural cure for cancer. The war on cancer falls within the framework of the current medical paradigm that tells us that medicine is on our side as they spend billions seeking elusive cures—while we all pay for it.

We live within a political paradigm where it is acceptable for private corporations and institutions to purchase laws that favor themselves and no one else. These laws are bought and paid for in the form of political contributions. If you ever want to know why big business can pollute our environment and dance away from lawsuits and any real taxes, just follow the money. The cross-pollination between private and public sectors in Washington, D.C. is at an all time high. Eli Lilly & Co., for example, mysteriously found its way into the Homeland Security Bill in November 2002. Buried within the bulky 450-page document was an outrageous clause that provides security to Eli Lilly & Co. from thousands of potential lawsuits against them by the families of autistic children who believe that their kids' condition is linked to thimerosal, a mercury-based preservative made by Eli Lilly & Co. that used to be a common ingredient in childhood vaccines. Currently, we are witnessing an autism epidemic. Where twenty years ago autism occurred in 1 of every 10,000 children, now it's more than 1 in 250. How did this mystery clause find its way into the Homeland Security Bill? No one knows. Or no one is talking. It took weeks to uncover the provision because it was secretly slipped into the bill sometime over the weekend before it was passed. Eli Lilly & Co. contributed $1.6 million in the last election cycle.

This type of deal-making goes on in Washington every day and affects everyone. Take mandatory vaccination, which is a policy that forces parents to buy some rich drug company's vaccine and inject it into their children or else face the consequences of their children not being enrolled in school. Forced vaccination is making drug companies rich. And, as always, this paradigm is held soundly in place through the masterful use of fear.

The current medical paradigm has taken on religious fervor over the last one hundred years, giving doctors an elevated, demigod status. For a time it was outlawed to heal cancer with any other means aside from surgery, chemotherapy, and radiation. Illegal! Many devoted doctors lost their licenses trying natural approaches to healing their clients. Many went underground with their therapies; some moved their research and clinics to other countries. Unfortunately, such arrogance has long overshadowed medicine—from the systematic destruction of midwives and herbalists during the time of witch-hunts to today's mandatory vaccination programs.

Before the hygiene paradigm, or rather lack of hygiene paradigm, was burst in the twentieth century with the discovery of microbes through greatly improved microscopes, doctors rarely washed their hands, or even their scalpels, between operations. One Hungarian doctor, Ignaz Semmelweiss, made the empirical observation that there was less incidence of death among expectant mothers and their new-borns in the ward where midwives were delivering than in the ward where doctors performed the deliveries. He traced this to the fact that midwives washed their hands before delivery and found that when he washed hands, especially after handling the dead, before delivering babies that the instance of childbed fever (epidemic at the time) declined dramatically and that the babies were healthier in general. He felt certain that washing his hands was reducing death and set out to prove his observations. He eagerly held meetings with other physicians to share his observation, but his fellow physicians laughed at him and reported his "ridiculous" theory to newspapers to scandalize him. Some doctors rebelled by wiping scalpels on the bottom of their shoe before operations. Clearly, Semmelweiss was coming from outside of a very well-protected hygiene paradigm that was fiercely defended by those solidly within it. After years of relentless public humiliation, Semmelweiss suffered a complete psychological breakdown and committed suicide, his message having fallen on deaf ears and his name having become the object of household jokes, even though he was correct in his observations. It took many years for this false paradigm to give way to an appreciation for hygiene. Today doctors wouldn't dream of not washing their hands between patients, and all surgical instruments are sterilized.

Hygiene is one of nature's favorite laws, one that is lavishly rewarded with good health. LifeFood Nutrition is extremely hygienic and creates a high degree of order inside the body. Nature is inherently wise; eating food in its freshest, whole form delivers this wisdom to the body. Munch on a freshly picked organic pear and the wisdom of an entire orchard is written within its highly ordered matrix. The DNA of the pear is written in nature's coded script. This script is easily read by the immune system for great efficiency in processing the pear.

It is true that we are what we eat, so keep it pure. You can become a keen observer of self-serving sales pitches by media and big business and use your own wise discernment in your choices of food and medicine. Health comes as we honor the simple and straightforward laws of nature and enjoy time-tested food and medicine that humans have consumed for thousands of years. Today it's more important than ever to be easy on the landfills by being modest with elaborately packaged food. During your life, what will you be casting off as you go? Microwave containers and tin cans, or avocado pits and pear cores?

ANNE PADDEN JUBB
Los Angeles, October 2003

CHAPTER 1

Foundations
of LifeFood Nutrition

The dust particles one can see silhouetted in a beam of sunlight, floating weightlessly through the air, are precursors to DNA, RNA, and life itself. Dust is the substance life is made of. These smallest imaginable insoluble minerals are extremely sensitive and respond to the vibration of universal energy. They are so small, in fact, that they possess Brownian Movement,[1] and dance to the cosmic and telluric forces of the universe. Life is made possible because of these colloids. These insoluble minerals exist in one of two forms, either in a colloidal state—invisibly small and suspended in liquid, gas, or gel—or in a solid state. When suspended in a fluid medium like blood, colloids of life exhibit an electrical charge that maintains an enormous amount of space around each of the components that make up the blood itself. If the charge is lost, colloids form into a solid, as the mineral colloids are attracted to each other. Colloid dust particles with the same electrical charge repel, while opposites attract. Colloids in this manner first crystallize, then coagulate, and finally congeal.

A good example of this process is a freshly made glass of juice, say a green drink like apple, celery, and kale. The fresh glass of juice is consistent in color—a bright green; it is closest to its whole living form. If left there for an hour you will see that the darkest green pigments will have settled to the bottom of the glass, while the juice at the top is rather transparent. What happened? As they separate, the apple, celery, and kale—from their whole essence to the processed (yes, the fiber is removed) juice—form electromagnetic energy drops and the juice separates. While the juice is fresh, the perky colloids are highly charged and invisibly small because they are evenly disbursed throughout the juice; however, as the electrical level drops, colloidal minerals that were repelled from each other only moments prior now become oppositely charged and cling to oppositely charged particles to become a solid (still very small) that settles to the bottom of the glass.

Life Is an Implosive Force

There are many forms of energy found in the universe, including hydraulic, sound, and electrical energy. However, there is a specific energy found in extraordinary healing that is known as radiant energy.[2] Colloidal biology utilizes radiant energy and provides an explanation of how to strengthen immunity and support the cellular structure that maintains health. This work stands on the shoulders of, and is supplemental to, our work in LifeFood Nutrition and tissue cleansing that is outlined in detail in the *LifeFood Recipe Book*,[3] most specifically in the unique way that we encourage saturating the body with electrolytes and colloidal vitamins and minerals (LifeFood) to target symptoms and heal them completely.

We understand that there only exists the disease of toxicity and enervation, which is a lack of electrical vitality at the cellular level, an overall lack of nerve force. LifeFood Nutrition increases blood and lymphatic flow that causes physiology to normalize. Familiarizing yourself with LifeFood Nutrition is crucial to understanding the depth of this work. The concepts are clearly outlined in the *LifeFood Recipe Book*, and rather than cover too much of the same territory here, we recommend you read it. At any rate, just so we are all on the same page, let's cover some of the foundations of LifeFood Nutrition.

A quick update: LifeFood Nutrition consists of fresh uncooked fruit and vegetable, soaked and sprouted nut and seed, fresh pressed oil, and some fermented food. We recommend organic and in-season fresh produce, or that it be properly dried and stored. LifeFood has its life force intact. It is vegetarian food from plants that can reproduce themselves in nature. It is sustainable agriculture that promotes shade, meaning grain, legumes, and all flesh food is omitted. Everything is prepared easy to digest: nothing is heated over 118° Fahrenheit to preserve the precious enzymes that the nutrient brings in naturally. We include whole food vitamin and mineral complex supplements, super food like spirulina, bee pollen, marine minerals, and goat whey, along with potent herbal remedies. LifeFood is a vegetarian diet that can include raw organic cheese (preferably goat).

Enzyme is LifeFood's buzzword. The enzymes in food have a survival temperature of 118° Fahrenheit. If whole food is cooked above and beyond that point, enzymes die. Enzymes digest our food for us. Enzymes must be there for digestion to occur. If food is without enzymes the body must scavenge from its personal supply to digest the nutrients our food supplies. This borrowing from important enzyme reserves within the body manifests as the process of aging. We witness the reversal of the process of aging within the first few days of beginning the LifeFood diet. Get out your blender because we recommend blending meals to get the most possible absorption of nutrients from the foods you consume. Fresh blended smoothies and soups, nutmilk and Electrolyte Lemonade (see recipes in *LifeFood Recipe Book*), are easy ways to get nutrition that require little digestive power from you. Uncooked blended meals contain super-powered vitamin and mineral colloids that mimic those found in the blood. This is the easiest way to digest and absorb these vitamins and minerals and make good use of the available nourishment. Most people in the modern world are digestively challenged. The Standard American Diet (SAD), consisting of sugar, starch (more sugar), rancid oil, and processed, denatured food, has taken its toll on the health and vitality of Americans and people the world over.

LifeFood Nutrition addresses the core foundation of life, advocating the consumption of nutrients that assist the running of a healthy immune system. Enzymes can be seen as the life force of food. Are enzymes present in your food, or will you be asking your body to dig into its reserves just so you can eat it? LifeFood is enzyme-packed to give you pure energy and cost you nothing. LifeFood digests itself. Enzymes are integral to all of the processes of the body. Uncooked food contains within it all the enzymes required to break food down. Of course, some uncooked foods are superior to others.

LifeFood is food that has a measurable life force. Life force is the property that allows something to be able to reproduce in nature. Life-Food is the food humans have biologically evolved to eat and digest. It is vegetarian and promotes shade over the land. LifeFood is vegetarian because animal flesh does not have life force.

Practicing the principles of LifeFood Nutrition is a way of being kind, gentle, and allowing with yourself and the Earth. It is the most sublime food humans can eat, and it also creates a sustainable future for the Earth. Wheat, corn, rice, carrots, beets, potatoes, bananas, dates, pineapples, and cane sugar do not contain much life force. This list of foods, though raw, cannot manage the chief undertakers—mold, fungus, and yeast. Cooked food is dead food that lacks a vital electrics and enzyme cache, forming colloids that become congealed and coagulated. Enzyme-resistant linkages form when food is cooked, making it become hydrophobic (water repellent).

LifeFood has a measurable force field made visible by Kirlean photography. The apple image on the cover of this book was taken with a Kirlean camera. You can witness the radiant living field of energy that surrounds the apple; this is the living matrix of the apple—a force that extends well beyond the apple's skin. This colorful radiant field surrounds all living things—trees, flowers, animals, and you. If you were to cook the apple and take another Kirlean picture, you would witness the disappearance of the spectacular color and range of light and electricity. Cooking food diminishes life force to the point that it can be completely dead, depending on how cooked or processed the food is.

Life is animated by electrical activity. It is important to consume food that has electrical activity and enzymes. Eating a diet rich in enzymes offers the body superior nutrition, complete with the electrical charge of life itself. Consuming a LifeFood diet, even a short time, provides experiential proof in itself as to how quickly the body heals when it is given the proper nourishment of whole food vitamins and minerals. The body is a perfect self-correcting mechanism. We are physical, emotional, spiritual creatures and health is a matrix of these factors that changes and fluctuates during the course of life.

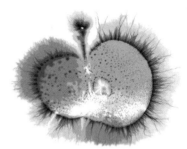

CHAPTER 2

Acid and Alkaline Body

Mold, Fungus, and Yeast Are
The Chief Undertakers of the Body

Trillions of platelets carried in the blood and lymph stream nourish every single cell by continuously quenching these structures with spare electrons. The maintenance of healthy tissue cells requires the proper amount of carbon dioxide, oxygen, and nutrition. Minerals in their colloidal form, as well as other nutrients, including sunlight, assist in promoting vessel dilation, which allows blood and lymphatic channels to be open and flowing. Everything works together synergistically; it is interesting to note that sunlight alone activates over two hundred enzymes into action. A true healing therapeutic incorporates knowledge of homeostasis, the physiological process by which the internal systems of the body, like blood pressure, body temperature, and acid-base balance, are maintained at equilibrium.[4]

The new science of colloidal biology is based on fundamental healing therapeutics, whereas allopathic medicine is not. Having a proper tissue and blood pH (a good acid/alkaline balance in the body) has been found to yield therapeutic effect in the body in four ways:

1) Maintaining enzymatic activity by generating the proper electrostatic valence for biochemical processes to occur;

2) Assisting biomechanics needed by the body due to states of stress or trauma;

3) Accelerating blood and lymph flow by maintaining cell metabolic activity and lysing and clearing away dead cellular and accumulated nu-toxic debris;

15

4) Enhancing immunity by presenting the body with nutrients in their most biologically available form.

BLOOD IS AN AMAZING JUICE truly understood only in regard to its relationship with the body as a whole. Blood sustains the entire body organ in nutrient delivery and waste management. Blood and life force have always stimulated human curiosity. Natural science has developed at a rapid pace, and along with it an interest in blood and the application of new emerging technology. We have now arrived at an understanding of blood formation and the role blood plays as an isotonic fluid[5] that supports life. Stunning leaps in the sophistication of microscopes over the last few decades offer a once hidden look within the human body. A universal order exists within us that is as vast and complex as one we gaze out at during the night. David and I have seen cells move with the application of blue and green fluorescent protein that makes individual parts visible under the microscope. We watched red blood cells fold and squeeze themselves into spaces and crevices as they would were they in the body.

Blood is an organ—a liquid organ. Blood streams through the vascular system, throughout the arteries, away from the heart to arterioles to capillaries, and returns via veins to the heart once again. Lymph, another fluid system we will examine later, involves managing the space between cells and clearing elements from between cells that would prevent them from otherwise fitting through the blood vessels.

Blood and lymph keep the body running beautifully. Both fluid systems are the first order of concern for those seeking vitality. Vitality is maintained as blood and lymph regulate the body much like a wet cell battery. Alkalinity causes a current and we have energy. When the battery is acidic, all spare electrons are expended. The body becomes low energy and degeneration sets in. The cause of much illness in the modern civilized world is due to the premature degradation of tissue (extreme acidity) and the body system through decomposition by bacteria, mold, fungus, and yeast. As long as the body has adequate oxygen and the body fluid and tissue have an acid/alkaline balance amazing health ensues. It's actually very simple.

A hidden cause of disease has to do with how the body handles hybridized and cooked denatured foods, especially acid-forming flesh, starch, and simple sugars that raise insulin. Acids and sugars rob calcium and other alkaline elements from the body. Foods that have colloids that are similar to mold, fungus, and yeast (i.e., foods stored in bins and silos) can be less than friendly on body chemistry. Flesh food generates putrefactive bacteria that will be housed within the intestinal tract. Eating fresh fruit and vegetables, easily digested, creates good internal hygiene, creating an environment for good clean blood.

Blood performs a great variety of functions in multi-celled organisms. Yet, single-celled organisms carry all their vital functions with them, the very same functions that multi-celled organisms do, such as transporting nutrients, the ability to reproduce, and the capacity for immune intelligence. Multi-celled organisms, however, have cells that are specialized to respond to the transmission of signals, movement, and other metabolic processes. The integrity of colloidal blood protein is vital such that fixed cells of the body that involve transportation, communication, and immunity are properly maintained to create vitality. Health challenges arise as an imbalance in the food we consume causes an undesirable interface within the body.

It seems that what we eat is more of a health factor than people have thought. Common reasoning is that there is a multitude of disease. Yet, David and I highlight the fact that keeping blood and body tissue at a proper pH keeps premature death at bay and makes the difference between vitality and death. This is the secret of an alkaline body.

If blood and lymph colloidal protein integrity is not optimal, fermentation may disturb the body's chemical bioelectric central homeostatic mechanism. A diet of refined starches and cooked denatured food can cause an over-acidification of body tissue, where the terrain of the very substance of self can ferment and/or putrefy.

Over-acidification of the tissue allows the terrain to support the proliferation of pleomorphic organisms.[6] What is it that occurs within five minutes of death that results in the coroner's never finding any endothelial cells[7] in the body? The answer to this question leads to an exciting understanding of biological transmutation[8] and helps explicate what wellness is. It's true that emotions like happiness or resentment, or the way one habitually frames their language and thoughts (either positively or negatively), affect acid/alkaline balance. However, the colloids of the food we eat and how close near those colloids are to biological transmutation into mold, fungus, or yeast is at the root of the etiology of all disease.

Tar, resin, and glue-like acid substance from cooked milk, grain, noodles, bread, pasta, and cooked flesh can cause adhesions (plaque) to plate and cause occlusion in blood vessels and lymphatic spaces, as well as adhesions in bile ducts and in and around the intestinal tract—gluing everything together.

MYCOTOXIN FROM MOLD, FUNGUS, and yeast can cause cells to be less receptive to LDLs[9] in the body serum. As that has happens, excess LDLs are disassembled by macrophage cells, which, after engulfing this debris, become a calcifying plaque that gradually lead to occlusion of blood vessels and other internal adhesions.

Enzymes Are pH Sensitive

Enzyme systems ensure that metabolism occurs as nature intended, and when they are not operating optimally, the body manifests its pathologies, which are the result of inefficient sugar, protein, and fat metabolism. People who die prematurely typically struggled with a metabolic challenge during their life. We understand that life begets life and dead begets dead. Cooked and denatured food leaves acid residue in the body and cooking food past 118° Fahrenheit diminishes essential enzymes. Only heat-resistant fermentive enzymes remain.

Enzymes require a specific pH. Enzymes biologically transmutate colloidal substrates and have very specific actions that involve an organized chain reaction and inextricable elemental forces. Thus, there are enzymes that can be secreted and extracted, and others that are fixed in the cell. Healing requires restoration of enzyme function in cancer and all pathological conditions.

Living cells radiate electrical potential into the space surrounding them. With its perfect positive and negative magnetic pole, each cell is a battery with its own measurable electrical emission, vibrating from every place throughout the body, from the open space of the stomach to the thyroid follicle, and beyond. Potassium is the intracellular colloidal ion and is electronegative in its surroundings, while sodium is biologically positive. Potassium likes to be near the positive nucleus and sodium likes to be near the alkaline extracellular fluid. These +/- colloidal ions provide us with the ability to propagate electrical potential across the cell membrane. Colloidal minerals activate enzyme systems.

Colloidal lithium, sodium, and calcium are biologically electropositive, while potassium sulfate, phosphate, and citrate are electronegative. The major electronegative center of the body is the thyroid. Because of its size, its amperage is small; yet, colloids give it a high voltage. Sodium can be deposited in the tissue of the thyroid and change its electromagnetic equilibrium, which is vital for homeostatic function. Colloids from salicylates (aspirin), sulfa drugs, thio-cyanates, and ionized calcium (mined from the ground, or from sea shells) can displace iodine from the thyroid.

Islets of Langerhans in the pancreas, bile capillaries, spleen, skin, and connective tissue make up the electronegative components of the body. Thyroid tissue is more alkaline than the brain! The thyroid and endocrine functions are often taxed when the body marshals immune responses to foreign protein, thus reinforcing the need for restoration of these vital systems. This is what the new science of colloidal biology is about. Organ vitality is integral in regulating the body's acid/alkaline balance.

Disease has a common biological root, which is results from morphological change in the tissue. The vitality of albumin/globulin ratio (to be discussed in later chapters) and reticuloendothelial[10] tissue integrity is important to good health. These are fragile cells, continuously being replaced, that line all passage ways including the stomach, colon, great glandular parenchymatous organs of the liver, pancreas, heart, blood vessels, and lymph passage ways. When the body is taxed with debris, endothelial cells function poorly.

Good immunity requires that the body get back its normal inflammatory response to foreign protein, which first requires tissue cleansing. This is the first step for people who are introduced to LifeFood Nutrition. We activate the organs of elimination. We advise our signature 14-Day LifeFood Nutritional Fast several times a year to liquefy stored material in the body and gently flush out overtaxed organs. This cleans up the blood very quickly, causing the whole body to look years younger and so electric and wholesome that it attracts comments from friends. Building good immunity is what colloidal biology and the secrets to an alkaline body is all about.

Mold and Yeast Recycle Life

There is a natural developmental cycle, originating from a very primitive stage, which has been identified as a microscopic colloid of life. Visible with a special microscope and only under certain lighting conditions, colloids can be seen aggregating into spores, then into bacteria and mold, hardening the cell wall and finally metamorphosing to culminate in a fungal and yeast form. Fungus and yeast are the culminating assent of the final developmental form of this primitive life cycle. Even the fibrin netting of clotting blood is a microbial form in its primitive stage that is activated in the blood. When the blood stops flowing, fibrin grows in vine-like netting as an automatic healing response.

What Is a Colloid (Kol oid)?

As a child I remember being fascinated by fine particles dancing in swirls through unseen currents of air illuminated by a beam of sunlight probing into the dark background of the room. These fine particles seen floating in the light of sunbeams are the very same colloids in the atmosphere that create the colors in a rainbow. Colloids are small and resist the pull of gravity, unless they are weighted down by moisture. The diamond sparkles of a dewdrop are the result of colloids of light.

All living things—even DNA itself—are made out of colloids of life. A colloid is a substance consisting of ultra-fine particles suspended in a medium, like an insoluble mineral suspended in water. Colloids are extremely tiny. Colloidal minerals are typically 0.01 to 0.001 microns in diameter. A billion of them can be put into a cube 400,000th of an inch small! Amazing! Some colloids are so small they're smaller than a visible wavelength of light, smaller than docosahexaenoic (DHA), a substance important in proper electrical patterning of the brain.

Colloids of life are imperishable, and at the end of human life the colloids we are composed of return to the earth to exist as colloids of life in the soil, where they can survive billions of years and eventually participate once again in consciousness. Colloids of life allow life to exist.

Brain cell membrane function occurs normally as long as DHA is present. Colloidal substrates get energy from DHA that come from omega-3 polyunsaturated fatty acids, such as flax seed and Brazil nuts. This helps protect and raise the electric tension of cells, resulting in more efficient use of oxygen while increasing cell absorption of nutrients. Colloids in the liver or kidneys of a healthy person are quite different from those in a less vital person.

A colloid that comes from lipoic acid is so small that it directly passes through the pores of the nuclear membrane and brings antioxidant protection to DNA. Colloids are the building blocks of DNA. Colloidal systems consist of insoluble particles of dissimilar ingredients that exist in solid, liquid, and gas states.

Colloids' insoluble, heterogeneous, and multiphasic properties interact to give colloids unique and fascinating characteristics that imbue themselves to life itself. Colloids of life make life possible! Particle colloids within a colloidal system are so small that they possess a field of energy that, if joined with other aggregates of colloids, give the assembled inanimate colloidal structure properties seemingly fitting of life.

Colloids and Bioelectric Resonance

Colloids of life from the great fission reaction of the sun and colloids of life from the earth compose all living things. Colloids of life are captured and stored by means of photosynthesis. Colloids of life from the celestial stars build and provide fuel for all living beings. There is an inexhaustible and free source of energy stored in cosmic rays on Earth—even in the middle of a blizzard. Plants and fruit tap into this energy. It is an energy drawn from the fission reaction of the celestial stars and the sun.

Cosmic energy, through increasing densification, forms the material we see in the universe. And someday, as time passes and this universe again becomes pure light, we will be able to regain our original nature. Cosmic energy travels from star to star in the heavens. Life is seemingly eternal. Life begets life. We also consider light, and that of which light is composed, to be eternal. Light just keeps traveling.

Photons are currently recognized as the smallest component of the sun's rays and are in perpetual and eternal motion. A photon can change its color (its frequency) depending upon how many of them are present. A photon is the purest form of energy, and when one unites with a second photon through resonance, they become a particle of a temporary nature.

Electrons capture energetic photons emitted from the fission of the sun through resonance. Electrons are made up of particles of elementary components of matter that are continuously in motion. Electron particles have their own wavelength with a particular oscillation and resonance—just like a radio receiver. As particles, they have their own length that in turn gives them their own frequency. Electrons are the final expression of matter, materialized as water in our bodies.

The material universe can be divided into two parts: *matter,* particles such as quarks, electrons, and muons; and *interactions,* such as gravity, magnetism, attraction, etc. Particles describe fields of one and a half integer-spin where only one particle can be in the same stage at any given time. Matter is divided into two categories: hadrons, which compose quarks; and leptons, which compose the remainder. Interactions are divided into four categories. They are listed in order of strength here: the strong nuclear force interacting with hadrons; electro-magnetism influencing charged hadrons and leptons; weak nuclear forces interacting with all hadrons and leptons; and gravity interacting with everything. Integer-spin is represented by particle interactions and is something other than the particle.

Many particles can exist in the same state. Gravity and electromagnetics interact on the grandest longest range from the farthest distance that you can imagine. Fields produced by matter in our universe add up and can be detected, even on a micro-scale.

Electrons orbit matter that consists of mostly the nucleus of the atom carrying a positive electrical charge. Electrons, in contrast, carry the negative charge. Both positive and negative attract because of opposing charges. Electrons exist in a space that is far away enough from their nucleus to ever be drawn away from their orbit. Electrons and photons love each other. Electrons attract photons through their magnetic field. As any electrical charge moves it emits a magnetic field.

Photons have a continuous magnetic field. As both electrons and photons have magnetic fields, they interact in resonance and their wavelengths are in tune; they attract to each other and the photon fits into the orbiting electron. Everything is actually caused as a result of resonance; everything is, in fact, resonance. Colloids have a resonance that results from its length. Colloids in seeds help organize and maintain life during the most critical steps of a plant's development. These are colloids of light, and are found in other life organisms where they perform a similar function.

An adult has approximately 9.55 pints (4½ liters) of blood. In a healthy person, blood is the fourth heaviest organ behind muscle, fat, and bone. Blood as a tissue is heavier than vital organs like the liver, heart, and brain. Lymph, of which lipoprotein is a major part, enters each heart chamber, and thus the blood, with each heartbeat. It is then percussed so that small lipoproteins cover every cell. This provides each cell with the most amazing antioxidant protection.

Colloidal lipoprotein coming from lymph enters the heart through the venous-laden blood on the right side, and oxygen-rich blood enters into the left heart chamber, creating a differential electrical potential. The distinct nutritive qualities coming into each chamber is important in generating the actual heart action potential. If the heart were without these colloidal lipoproteins as essential fatty acids the heart muscle would become cytochrome oxidase deficient.

Under an electron microscope a major distinguishing feature of a cancer cell is the presence of visible fat in its cell nucleus membrane cytoplasm. Cooked fat is dead and does not transmit electricity efficiently; it insulates instead. The presence of isolated fat in cancer cells and rheumatic muscle cells is a telling observation.

Food with added preservatives cause respiration poisoning that obstructs cell metabolism of lipids (fats). Our body's mucus membrane needs highly unsaturated fats made from intestinal flora when we are healthy. We can also get it from fresh food. It may come as a surprise that part of the etiology of diabetes and many other conditions, is actually a compromised ability to metabolize fat.

In an alkaline body there are spare electrons, and having spare electrons equals having a long life. Cis-unsaturated fatty acids[11] give us bipolarity so the wet cell battery within us has a current. Trans-fatty acids are dead fat. We need both poles of the battery to get a current. If one pole is disconnected the current loses the ability to flow. Our ability to cope with stress depends largely upon this battery's ability to continually recharge.

Unsaturated fats (EFAs) are important in colloidal biology and the secrets of an alkaline body because they have an abundance of spare electrons. Growth can become impaired and disturbed if unsaturated fatty acids are missing because of our need for both electrical poles to function.

Active lipids are needed in the surface membrane of red blood cells to keep their membranes electrically negative, thus, blood cells are kept restrained from each other, allowing for greater cell respiration and waste removal in the body. Otherwise, the surface membrane is inefficient in its exchange of nutrient and waste material within the body. Heat-processed oils and fresh fish oils are rancid and toxic and composed of trans-fatty acid; they should be avoided in human nutrition. Trans-fat cannot be processed by the body for integration into living tissue. A sulfur-bearing amino acid, such as cystine, has a positive electric charge and is an excellent lipotropic protein combination. Cystine, found in nuts, is capable of making unsaturated plant fats soluble. All cooked fat, and pig fat especially, is unable to combine with water, causing it to separate out and be stored in the body. Cooked fats are not miscible with water so they travel separately making blood sluggish, and eventually being stored.

Lipids becomes water soluble when surrounded by proteinaceous colloids that become carrying units as lipoproteins. Unsaturated fat is rich in electrons and causes very high cell surface capillary activity. The further you go into the atom the denser it gets, whereas the more you move out of the atom, in the direction of electrons, the lighter and less dense the matter gets.

Blood, the juice of life, is an isotonic fluid because of its high electron-rich nutrition. Blood and body serum can move through the tiniest places, penetrating the furthest reaches within us. Electron-rich nutrients are needed for proper capillary activity for lymph, blood, and the mucus membrane for proper elimination to occur.

Electrons Are Light Matter

Electrons have a high affinity for oxygen, which is why they crowd to the surface, thus stimulating cell respiration and keeping the delicate balance of the electrically negative cell membrane and its positive nucleus within. One can thrive on half the normal intake of food as long as we consume high electron-rich nutrients.

Sexual and fertility function are dependant upon the important relationship between fat and protein. In men, sperm has one thousand times more sulfur-rich protein than any other cell in the body, while in women lecithin and unsaturated fat abound in the female ovum.

The more alive something is, the more it is moving from the dense matter of nucleons and protons to the world of light and electrons. Having an abundant supply of electrons increases vitality. When a bird dies from having ingested a pesticide/insecticide-laden life form it is because that environmental toxin challenged the bird's electrons' ability to remain in harmony. Interestingly, this challenge did not affect the more primitive life form—the insect.

Simple-celled organisms living in symbiotic and dysbiotic relationships within our intestinal tract become completely poisoned when an antibiotic is used. The vagus nerve that enervates the stomach and intestinal tract is a parasympathetic nerve, which, if pinched would cause acid residue. This can affect the liver, heart, lungs, stomach, pancreas, intestine, thyroid, gonads, and primitive part of the brain stem.

A hidden cause of disease is the consumption of dead, refined, and denatured food. These types of food deplete alkaline reserves of potassium, magnesium, iron, and calcium from the body because they mostly turn to alcohol. Alcohol produced from the fermentation of dead food is pure liquid yeast. A major ionization is needed to neutralize acid deposited in the body from lavish living. Lavish living causes us to leech anionic elements like calcium that is found in food sources having grown toward the sunlight, such as dark leafy green vegetables, and all food that grows its fruit above ground on vines, branches and bushes. Precious anionic elements are sorely needed in most health conditions. A vital body equals having spare electrons. Blood and lymph are isotonic fluids[12] because colloids have spare electrons that keep colloidal protein unobstructed and flowing.

From Dust We Come and to Dust We Return

Life colloids are simple life forms that exist in many forms, from assemblages of colloids of life (somatids)[13] to single-celled organisms. Life colloids such as phytoplankton, billions of years old, that are placed in a fluid medium can get busy, come to life, and change their genetic code to survive—more rapidly than anyone thought! Seemingly, genetics is more functionally plastic for simple life forms than we knew.

You may be surprised to learn how many simple life colloids we are composed of. If we only look at the more simple intermediary life colloids like bacteria, and we leave out the more evolved forms like mold, fungus, and yeast, an adult has more than four hundred species of bacteria in their body—exceeding the count of cells in the body by ten- to one hundred-fold! These primitive life colloids provide us with nourishment and protection, allowing for symbiosis to occur. This is a rich inner world full of mystery and inherent wisdom. It's become evident that colon bacteria even communicate with intestinal epithelial cells to call forth needed nutrients.

Colloids assemble into larger, more complex organisms from the incorporated colloidal structure of a more primitive life. That is, primitive organisms (life colloids) are a collection of colloidal minerals that are formed from both simple to more complex structures. The fully assembled life colloid structure is the result of a morphogenic[14] pattern instilled within the terrain of the colloids that cause all characteristic life forms to materialize. A morphogenic pattern is the intelligent blueprint energy field matter uses to assemble itself. One example is the morphogenic field that creates a seed and holds all the information that seed needs to grow into a tree, and the trees into orchards.

Imagine the tiniest grains of sand on a thin membrane, like a drum-head, and a sound directed to it that causes the fine grains of sand and the membrane to resonate. Were you to witness this firsthand you might be surprised to see a fish or a butterfly or a person's face appear among the particles of dancing grain. All shapes of life appear as the grains vibrating on this thin membrane and assemble into familiar forms created by the sound wave being emitted.

CHAPTER 3

The New Science
of Colloidal Biology

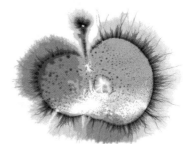

A Morphogenic Field Assembles Life Colloids

Atoms have a corresponding synergistic field that has a standing wave form in which its frequency and amplitude control what the structure looks like. What something looks like on the outside is a result of the transform of these waves of energy inside. Though we begin life symmetrically, small instabilities build to develop a stable asymmetrical form. The base material congregates at vibrational standing points that, depending upon rotational movement, cause unique- and characteristic-shaped spaces to form as major eddies of energy activity. The visible physical appearance of things is the inverse of the invisible vibration within.

Photons of violet light are an energy coming toward and infrared waves are traveling away. Photons are electrons that exist as a harmonic of the same waveform. All matter is essentially waves of resonance. Harmonics dislodge electrons in a photoelectric effect. Violet light does this, as it is a powerful short wavelength.

Gravity and radio waves are perceivable only because of their effect on phenomena. Let's imagine this morphogenic field in action. It is dramatically illustrated in the activities of the humble earthworm. The earthworm, so well appreciated we gave it the name of our planet and soil, possesses amazing regeneration abilities. When the earthworm is cut in two the tail end of the worm's intestinal tract becomes active as residual earth travels downward and remains at the bottom of the tract. While this is happening the wound becomes clean and red. It's interesting to note that throughout this process, it's been shown that the earthworm's tail end always remembers which direction is forward. Earthworms receive information from their severed top halves because identical DNA emits a transform of energy that enables the tail end to completely regrow a new brain, mouth, and digestive apparatus, as well as five new hearts! The tail end of the original earthworm becomes a clone. Regeneration occurs from the material of the clot as the colloids assemble into the morphogenic pattern imbued in the terrain surrounding these colloids.

Tiny flatworms called planarians, careful to avoid the light, regenerate their whole bodies after having fasted to nearly nothing. These common species of flatworms completely regenerate a brand new head. Full mature sea sponges disassemble into many small pieces and then regenerate from these tiny clumps back into mature sponges. This understanding of morphogenic fields has led us to an understanding about the communicative capability within a cell that transmits information to other cells. Our cells can still communicate without needing to be directly connected, but through this morphogenic resonance that is emitted and received by other cells as radio waves. Colloids from simple life colloids, to life colloids as cells, to entire whole bodies, emit personalized call signs that are an instant direct connection as a field of primary perception.

Compared to deeper tissue, a skin cell is impervious to ultraviolet radiation. The bark or skin of the plant covers the entire plant except its growing root tip, which is where growth hormone is released in the dark. Root tips are light sensitive. Blue light emitted from within the plant is what guides the assemblage of colloids to form into the root from the cytoplasm of life colloids in the soil. In the same way, our skin provides an electromagnetic waveform guide that protects cells so intercellular communication occurs in an orderly fashion. A similar waveform guide exists in the plant at the root tip, allowing for growth and cellular replication to occur at this site.

Electromagnetic waveform principles, such as those in homeopathy[15] or sacred geometry,[16] allow us to see quinine's effect on malaria. On an electromagnetic level the herb quinine has the same waveform frequency as malaria. The effect of one over the other illustrates a principle of homeopathy, where two same waveforms within a system annihilate each other. Universal principles can be observed in nature. Atmospheric electricity collects in points and spires, facilitating an ion exchange between earth and sky. There are reservoirs deep within us that are in resonance with celestial energy from the farthest reaches of outer space. Enormous fission reactors occurring in the celestial stars and sun provide the body with potential energy that can be tapped.

As long as your heart and brain waves are coherently in tune you are a perfect instrument for divining. There is a direct semiconductive current that is flowing along insulation material of nerves and connective tissue in your body. Waveforms, even as thoughts and feelings impinging upon the flux of this antenna, can be selectively culled by the brain. Enormous amounts of information are transmitted through radio waves. Through resonance, energy is sent without any physical connection necessary at all.

The Morphogenic Field of Conception

The body's developed morphogenic field involves nerve junctions on either side of the spine, which create electromagnetic oscillation. Dipole fields arise from the brain's nerve structure and axons in the spinal cord. The oscillatory and polarizing energetics of a morphogenic field cause colloids to assemble into the myriad of organic and inorganic structures. Lower and higher velocities of conduction cause the forming organic structure to have either wide and less differentiated dispersion, or an elongated ovum shape, respectively. The combination of elements provides a code that determines all aspects of our form. This includes a morphogenic resonance that emits from all like structures in existence that causes a niche to occur for each species of life on Earth. Each species has a niche, or place, within the over-all holographic matrix of the planet itself. When a species becomes extinct, such as the saber-tooth tiger, their niche ceases and the morphogenic resonance of the species reconstructs, or morphs, into other life forms within the nested layers of geometry that make up the Earth's matrix.

Explained through sacred geometry, all of the knowledge of the universe is brought together when the sperm and ovum join to form a vesica piscis. The sperm and ovum have passed into each other to form the first cell. Simple organisms evolved into cells. Let's discuss in simplistic terms how we are created from parents. At conception, the energetics of male and female pronuclei from the parents join to become a vesica piscis that is the nuclei of the first human cell, called a zygote. Mitosis[17] of the zygote occurs when the positive and negative poles form as a tube of colloids that, interestingly, is always in perfect alignment with the north and south poles of the Earth.

At the exact moment of conception, there is a perfect symmetry, as witnessed in sacred geometry. The first cell contains the knowledge of itself and another cell; an organism of two cells has the knowledge of itself and two more, making four cells. Four cells form a cube (a tetrahedron) that has the knowledge to bring forward four more—to total eight—cells (a star tetrahedron, also a cube). These original first eight cells that form us are different than any other cells that we will form during our lives. It is said that these original cells are immortal and that while every other cell will die and be replaced by a new one, these original eight will remain. They are with us until we die. These eight identical original immortal cells reside at the exact geographic center of our body (just above the perineum). From these eight cells we grow radically outward. The original eight cells instantly double to become sixteen (a cube within a cube). We grow asymmetrically from this point onward. The forming embryo becomes a hollow sphere (tube torus), one end becoming the mouth and the other the anus. It's interesting to note that from this moment forward primitive life colloids (spores, double spores, and endoblastic cells) play a vital role in protecting the child from the mother's immune system.

Primitive Life Spontaneously Arises

Nature is replete with examples of spontaneous generation, such as simple-celled organisms like bacteria arising out of putrefying blood and other protein-rich material. Simple life forms are everywhere and have even been found in meteorites from outer space. Colloids of life arise from phytoplankton; all life is built from cosmic energy being condensed. The colloids of these primitive life forms become incorporated into larger-celled organisms. A cell originally arises out of a place where there was not one previously! Cells arise from simple colloidal protein substrate, such as in the colloids of an egg. One red blood cell arises in the egg without a single cell having existed there prior. It just appears out of nowhere, or rather, out of the substrate of the egg. We also know that bacteria will spontaneously arise from rotting protein and that even pasteurized urine can become turbid. Primitive life spontaneously arises out of the colloids of life that then go on to join together to make proteins. This is the building material of life.

Red blood cells arise from the colloidal substrate the food we eat. The substrate colloids of blood become incorporated into cells of our body and other organisms, both symbiotic and dysbiotic. Colloids have arrived from other organisms and are the building blocks that compose the cells that make up the tissue of the heart, ears, eyes, and every other part of the body. Organs, and even the clotting factor in blood, are aggregates of symbiotic organisms made of life colloids. These aggregates, living in symbiotic relationship, are what make up larger organisms. The liver is composed of life colloids similar to the Kombucha mushroom (see recipe in Appendix).

Colloidal biology is the result of an exciting observation and study of the behavior and function of living substrates, including red blood cells of amphibians, birds, and mammals through histological section and dark and bright phase contrast microscopic investigation. It is interesting to note from these studies that mitotic cell division[18] in the muscles, adipose tissue, bone marrow, and liver show extremely low values. Mitotic cell division figures do not account for cell proliferation, whereas colloidal biology fills in the gaps and offers a fresh new look at how and where red blood cells are most commonly formed.

Extra-vascular red blood cells (erythrocytes) that are scattered between various tissues are a collection of colloids that are easily seen in transition, assembling into various tissues depending on the degree of health of the cellular terrain. This is regenerative tissue that acts by transforming a pool of colloids, comprised of disintegrating red blood cells and plasma proteins as a colloidal cache (monera) toward the synthesis of DNA, into lymphocytoid or mesenchymal cells!

Orthodox medicine has other than done a good job of considering the information available as its practitioners have been stuck in an old paradigm. Though there is an uncritical acceptance of the orthodox theory of cell proliferation, this theory is challenged by a large body of information bearing on the production of blood cells and platelets and their lifecycles (hemopoiesis), and the behavior of oxygen-toting red blood cells (erythrocytes) in humans. There are questions that bear contemplation: How does the hemocytoblast[19] arrive and proliferate? How does the denucleation of the normoblast[20] occur since red blood cells are without a nucleus? What happens to the cells in the bone marrow that apparently make the blood? What is the relationship between coagulation of the blood and erythrocytes? What happens to the red blood cell when it is spent as a gas transporter? What is the relationship between red blood cells and white blood cells? The orthodox theory of cell proliferation as it regards all of these matters is being challenged by ongoing scientific discovery and the concepts of colloidal biology.

It is widely held in conventional medicine that the red blood cell is the most highly differentiated cell and that it multiples through mitotic division of cells primarily in bone marrow. It posits that the red blood cell is simply an oxygen and carbon dioxide transporter that degenerates after 90 to 120 days. However, it's important to point out that hemocytoblasts arise from certain protein-rich organic substrates where cells do not exist before. Examples in nature abound of cells freely arising, such as the embryonic villi yoke sack inside an egg; colloidal caches (monera) derived from spent red blood cells, and from the monera of the digested substrate colloids within the villi of the intestine.

Reversible differentiation of fatty tissue into red blood cells occurs as the body goes into a state of autolysis during fasting conditions! Furthermore, we can witness bacteria arise spontaneously from putrefying organic matter. In the ocean, we know that cells arise in coral and sponge from aggregates of intracellular symbionts in the water—aggregates that fuse together and organize themselves.

The colloids of red blood cells have been seen extruding, and in some cases adhering and fusing with colloids in the body serum. The colloids of the erythrocyte in vitro have been seen assembling themselves into bell-shaped and constricted forms, which ultimately transform into a spherical form (spherocyte). Throughout this process the collected colloids' surface area can display a heaving and contracting wavelike movement because of the property of Brownian motion. Colloids of the extruded cytoplasm of disassembled red blood cells join into strings and display an active rotating motion. Once the round-cell spherocyte forms, it can become a number of things, including a white blood cell (leukocyte) or other simple life form depending upon the integrity of the morphogenic terrain from which the cache of colloids formed.

All life colloids and larger organisms first arise from the formative forces of water upon the firmament being expressed as electrical attractions and as assemblages of mineral colloids. All animal life as we know it has sodium chloride in its extracellular fluid which reveals that we evolved from the sea; plants, on the other hand, have potassium and evolved out of the land. This relationship of plants to animal life involves a consciousness between fatty acids and hormones (sterols).

If you look at a lump of humic shale under a microscope, what is normally invisible appears to be living because it is moving. Humic shale is a deposit of organic minerals from plants that lived thousands of years ago. In just one hundred grams there can be several million life colloids (ferments) of infinitesimal size and of immense antiquity.

These colloids are also found in mineral water, soil, slime marshes, and in decomposing organic matter.

Colloids of Life

Moving particles in the soil, living blood, fermenting hay, cell cultures, ferments, and living tissue have been observed through microscopes for more than one hundred years. Tiny spear-, corkscrew-, and other-shaped particles have had many names over the past century: centrioles, plastids, vacuoles, granules, filaments, fibrilles, ferments, microzymes, bions, BX virus, protids, cryptocide progenitors, somatids, and now colloids of life. All life arises out of a symbiotic relationship between microscopic colloids of life that form into life colloids. Colloids of life are the substrate material of our body.

Colloids of life, such as microorganisms and cells, are assembled from minute mineral colloidal particles, which, because of their small size, pick up cosmic energy from the way they spin and their possession of Brownian movement. Colloids from fruit, and those of a mountain stream, pick up quite a bit of energy that is imbued into a fluid, giving it a zeta potential.[21] These minute minerals have an electrical charge that keeps them in perpetual motion within a fluid medium. The atoms within these minute minerals can gain or lose electrons, taking on either a negative charge (anionic-alkaline) or a positive charge (cationic-acidic) as a result.

Enzymes are the agents of colloidal nutrition. They depend upon an activation (anabolic or catabolic) of a specific level of consciousness that is a merging between levels of mineral, plant, and animal consciousness through the process of biological transmutation. Enzymes work within a specific acid/alkaline pH balance. Life colloids must maintain proper potassium levels inside their membranes relative to sodium levels outside, since electrons flow toward the positive pole. Altering this latter relationship compromises health. A proper balance of positively charged to negatively charged ions is important for the expression of life.

An Ion is an atom that has gained or lost an electron. A small percent of the ions occur from a discreet few water molecules. Yet, this very small percent is necessary for many metabolic precesses occur only as ions are present. Water is medium where chemical reaction takes place. Water is a universal solvent due its available protons and electrons.

Colloids of life are found in the water of living things. A colloid of life is a tiny particle in a colloidal dispersion. A colloid of life has a charged nucleus with ions surrounding it. Water imbued with colloid of life catalyzes its molecules that join into strings. These strings (about .04 inch) are visible under a microscope. Colloids of life assist all life structures to gather water.

Water of life has unique structure involving the colloid of life structuring the molecules so they join into .04 inch long strings. Regular tap and bottled water is without colloids of life that structure water into strings. These colloids of life cause a slight attraction between molecules that raises the surface tension of water. These colloids of life allow water to be slightly in a structured state as a liquid crystal. Water on the inside of a cell has a beautiful colloidal lattice structure

Water on the inside of a cell has a beautiful colloidal lattice structure. This lattice structure among other things allows for ions and other elements inside the cell. This lattice structure inside is responsible for a magnoelectrics vital for cell functioning.

Magnetism is a field of energy given off around an electrical current that is flowing. Life directly applies this magnetic field. Electromagnetic baths all life as the condensed effects of cosmic energy. Colloids of life and life colloids collect, store and apply this energy to pump disorder out. This current is only about a billionth of an amp. A colloid of life is a condenser that draws free electrons from the air and water of its surrounds. The colloid of life is able to do this because of its structure.

Colloids of life have an enormous negative surface charge. A Colloid of life attracts the positive end of a water molecule. In this way the colloid of life attracts strings of water molecules around itself. This veil of water molecules that the life colloid had around itself attracts a fresh source of spare electrons that are engaged in all life chemical reactions.

The electromagnetic filed allows water molecules present to contribute electrons and protons into biological and chemical transmutation of one element into another.

Water molecules that surround the colloid of life are a ready supply of protons and electrons. These water molecules joined into strings that surround the colloid of life allows the colloid of life to act as a condenser. This effect is what gives the body a current. Colloids of life collect and attract electrons from water and air.

Attracting to the positive end of a hydrogen bond, the colloid of life's extremely powerful negative surface valance causes other molecules of water to have also become strung together . A reticular magnetic field flows from the water clathrates in these short strings that form around a colloid of life. The water surrounding the colloids of life become harmonically orchestrated in a manner where cosmic energy is taped from the cosmos.

Colloids of life are the building blocks of DNA and can hold water close to themselves in such a way that this becomes an available source of protons and electrons. Energy is liberated from the transmutation of the water molecules that are held close to the Colloids of life. This energy enables the life colloid to pump this disorder out of itself. The water molecules immediately adjoining the colloid of life are biologically transmutated into elements required by the life colloids.

Colloids of life assemble into life colloids that are the greatest alchemical life forms on the planet. This can be seen as a bio-diverse biological mat of Colloids of life assembled into life colloids. Life is composed as a multitude of these life forms living in harmony with each other.

Colloids of Life can harness water and this energy can be applied by the life form to reduce activated oxygen and all myriad of the life forms tasks where energy is required. Life Colloids can act as a powerful antioxidant increasing the life forms ability to maintain self.

Colloids of Life assemble life water and life manner. Most elements are found with energy levels unfulfilled. Hydrogen is the most abundant element in the universe (more than 90 percent of all matter) and it is predominantly found without its electrons. Some elements are inert and others are hungry for their energy fields to be complete. Reactive compounds formed require energy to be reduced.

Colloids of life love to have enough spare electrons. Colloids of life and life colloids act as a catalyst that assists the life form to maintain itself by taping zero point energetic (ZPE).

These tiny strings of water .04 of an inch long are applied in maintaining a cells inner water structure. The structure of a cell is composed of colloids of life and life colloids that have their own DNA and reproductive schedule. Colloids of life replenish their requirement for electrons and electrons. Life can gain or lose electrons.

Colloids of life act as catalysts in biological transmutations of one element into another. Colloids of life emit their effect through this structured water that surrounds them. This enables colloids of life to effect a variety of reactions because:

A. Colloids of life possess vacuum energetics by their enormous surface area charged negatively that causes water molecules to be attracted.

B. Colloids of life as condensers that emit a reticular magnetic effect that allows it to provide electrons for alchemical biological transmutation.

C. Colloids of life tap water and air for vitally needed protons and electrons applied in the chemistry of life.

Colloids of life structure water and assist with electromagnetic effects. Carbon bonded to four other carbon molecules creates a diamond. If only three carbon molecules bond graphite is the result. In a similar way, colloids of life change the shape of how water molecules crystalize when frozen and in their expanded light state.

A Clathrate can be found in the very thin film of water that covers all things that are little hollow spheres of water molecules. These hemispheres? Get as condensers and transmitters of energy through resonance emitted reticular magnoelectrics.

Life water is heavy hydrogen deuterium.

Life manner is carbon formed from colloids of life transmuting hydrogen into carbon ZPE (zero-point energetics is about tapping free energy.

Catalyst is an agent that assists speed up a reaction yet is other than used itself.

Biological Water Is Living

The cells in your finger have the same DNA as those in your ear. Cells that have identical DNA become specialized as a result of the morphogenic field present within you. Damaged cells regenerate and new ones grow to regain the original configuration of the healed body part. The moment this is complete the repair process ceases. Our morphogenic field is a localized intelligence that reverts us to normal as quickly as possible.

Water makes up the larger percentage of our body averaging about ten gallons. Water and lymph act more often like a gas than a liquid inside us. They can penetrate right through us, even through the dentin of the teeth. Ninety percent of blood is water. Water has amazing properties. It is lighter as it becomes more solid. Water is the most important solvent on the planet, and it is living!

Water is one oxygen atom that has two small hydrogen atoms sticking to it like Micky Mouse ears—the ears being hydrogen. Sometimes they cluster at one end of the oxygen molecule, making that end positive and the other end negative. Water is so alive that the hydrogen atoms slip from one end of the oxygen atom to the other continuously in a uniform way at a rate of 10^{11}/second. Often, the bonding angle for water is $104.5°$ Fahrenheit in a liquid state and $109.5°$ Fahrenheit when solid. The bonding angle is more open when water is frozen (solid), and also when water is more structured. The water in blood is very highly structured.

Water molecules join to make hexagonal to pentagonal shapes. Water is layered as it is bound to protein. The first layer is fixed more to the protein substrates. The layer furthest out is called bulk water, the layer in between is called the interface layer. Enzymes interact in the interface layer. This water has a lower freezing point at -10° Celsius. Sixty-four percent of this interface layer is mostly hexagonal-shaped water structures, the same shape as snow. The interface layer is therefore the best layer of water for plankton and algae to grow in because it is so highly structured.

Healthy body tissue has this structured interface layer of water, while malignant tissue lacks it. Hexagonal-shaped water structure is found around ionized calcium. Ionization is a process that can occur naturally in water, called electrolytes. Ionization happens in the body as oxygen and hydrogen atoms gain or lose electrons, making them electrically charged and therefore more chemically active. Ionized water splits in half. One half is the H+ ion (acid), the other the hydroxel ion OH- (alkaline). The concentration of these two ions in relationship to each other in the body brings about enzyme homeostasis and life as we know it. Life begets life and dead begets dead.

Alkaline Forming Elements	*Acid Forming Elements*
potassium (K)	sulfur (S)
sodium (Na)	phosphorus (P)
calcium (Ca)	chlorine (Ch)
magnesium (Mg)	iodine (I)
iron (Fe)	

Colloidal Isotonic Proteins Bathe Cells

A vertebrate is composed of cells, bathed in a fluid that is similar to seawater, composed of a lipo-proteinacious ground substance. This ground substance, carried by all vertebrates, bathes the cells in the body. Inside an adult human, this fluid consists of some forty liters of slightly sweet saline solution that must maintain a proper level of acid/alkaline homeostasis/hygiene. This watery ground substance is the basis of particle colloids, proteins, fats, muco-poly saccharides, high-density lipoprotein, and neuro-immunological substrates that bathe cells and bring nutrients along. Blood pH plays a major role in the biological transmutation of toxins, as well as the tagging, clearing, and removal of waste material from cell metabolism and other dysbiotic life forms. This state of radiant health is achieved in a terrain where cells have a pH of 6.8 and blood has a pH of 7.3.

Fine protein-derived colloid particles make it into the brain through the blood-brain barrier. The ability to combine protein and fat in the body is very important for longevity and maintaining proper hygiene. Most people believe that blood simply remains within the capillaries and veins. Most acclaimed authorities haven't the foggiest idea as to how blood is actually formed. Under certain conditions a large array of protein-derived particles, small enough to pass through tiny openings of the capillaries, passes through into the lymphatic system. Red blood cells can also squeeze and pass through into the space between cells. Under certain conditions even fibrin, albumin, and globulin can pass through this space between cells. This watery ground substance bathes our cells and brings spare electrons into, and oxidized cell waste out of, the cells. Management of this system is another secret of an alkaline body.

Our body systems must maintain the homeostasis of this protein-derived ground substance of our blood plasma. Small-particle colloids, mostly made of protein and fat (high-density lipoprotein), carry nutrients to the furthest places in the body. The assimilation area in our body responsible for combining protein and fat must be kept clear and open. Proper ingredients are needed to assemble high-density lipoprotein (HDL) and low-density lipoprotein (LDL). LDLs transport nutrient *away* from the liver, while HDLs transport lipids and fat *back* to the liver. This keeps the proper pH balance; inside the cell at a pH of 6.8, and the outside watery ground substance that bathes the cells at a pH of 7.35.

Most people who eat modern denatured food are constipated. It's not uncommon for David and I in our work to meet people who have only one bowel movement a week, if they're lucky. The intestine has to be kept moving with a robust peristalsis. Stored toxins have to be neutralized for proper health to be maintained. There are many factors to consider in maintaining the colloidal integrity of the body, like acid/alkaline balance and having plasma colloidal protein integrity. A proper blood profile is important in the restoration of other body systems.

Breathing Changes pH of Blood

B reathing is by far one of the most important acid/alkaline buffers. A couple million years ago our atmosphere was 30 percent carbon dioxide; today it is .035 percent. The alveoli of our lungs are designed to maintain excellent oxidative metabolism through proper oxygen to carbon dioxide ratio.

Our breath is a major factor in changing this acid/alkaline balance. A person's body, though young, may die unexpectedly. A person who was seemingly healthy one day, vibrant and full of electricity, may experience a state of weakness and debilitation the next.

Many conditions such as strokes, embolisms, aneurysms, heart attacks, and a variety of other ailments and life threatening conditions occur most often between the hours of 4 A.M. to 10 P.M. What is it about these times that cause the body system's architecture and functioning to be challenged? A critical factor is how much carbon dioxide the body retains. This relates to good oxygenation of the body. Proper oxygenation of the body requires carbon dioxide. Carbon dioxide is a smooth muscle dilator.

Relaxed, quiet, and still breathing causes the alveoli to continuously trap carbon dioxide-causing carbonic acid, raising the acidity of the erythrocytes (red blood cells) and bringing healthy oxygenation throughout the whole body. People may be surprised to learn that carbon dioxide causes the red blood cells to have a good carbon dioxide/

oxygen dissociation curve. This means that the blood has excellent ability to release its oxygen; otherwise free radicals and active oxygen can cause sedimentation and crystallization of colloids in our connective tissue that brings about a hardening of connective tissue and vascular and neural tissue contraction and sclerosis.

Unchecked inflammation is the sign of a compromised immune system, and is often accompanied by a wasting of body tissue, caused by a leaky gut and immune complex-laden plasma that arise in this environment. In a cleansed body, immune cells become educated as to what is *self* and what is *other.* In this way, dendritic cells, imbedded in between cells, sample the terrain to identify toxins and alert immune cells. In an immune-compromised body, dendritic cells don't expose themselves and as a result immune cells aren't programmed to respond properly.

We maintain the proper acid/alkaline carbon dioxide/oxygen equilibrium in our blood through calm, full, quiet nose breathing. Nose breathing is an important habit for us to practice and maintain to ensure a properly vital, rich source of electrons and protons as ground substance for bathing our cells. This includes maintaining everything in our blood, including somatids, spores, double spores, red and white blood cells, and plasma proteins, in a healthy ratio. Otherwise, too many red blood cells, white blood cells, globulins, fibrins, and foreign proteins take up all the space, causing important elements like albumin, the super transporter, to be unavailable for water and other nutrients to be transported to places in between cells.

Our breath brings life to cells. Robust, deep breath oxygenates the whole system, which is so important for the brain. Oxygen and fat are the primary fuel sources for the brain. A very important adaptation for our times is in the way we breathe. Do you breathe through your nose when you sleep? Breathing through your nose during sleep, and also during waking hours, is very important. Ideas come to us during the inspiration (inhalation) through our nose.

Proper breath, and other habits of internal and external hygiene, allows body fluids to functionally hydrate cells. As long as the body is hydrated, the connective tissue will maintain a youthful essence. Hydrated cells, which can literally be twice as hydrated as dehydrated cells, give a person a youthful look.

Colloidal Protein in Evolution

Throughout time there have been great changes on the Earth that have caused us to continually change and adapt. Climate changes, migration, floods, war, famine, earthquakes, volcanoes, and good old fashioned curiosity have moved us across the globe to set up residence in nearly every region and adapt to its environment and food sources. Environment and food sources have quite a lot to do with how our physical appearance can change over the generations. You might smile looking at a suit of armor from the Middle Ages, to see how much larger we've become over many hundreds of years, especially in America where commercial bird and animal flesh is laden with steroids and gigantism is on the rise. All things are in a constant state of change. Some changes are very fast and some are so slow you'd have to live a thousand years to notice them. You can find seashell fossils in rocks on the top of the Rocky Mountains, a living record of past centuries of shifting ocean levels and terrain. Indications on the rocks mark a time when an enormous amount of water once lapped at the top of these newly forming mountains. You can find the entombed trunks of ancient trees hidden deep below the surface of modern mountain lakes.

Humans, along with a few other primates, have spent time evolving very rapidly through a semi-aquatic environment. Between 12 million and 3.7 million years ago, our ancestors indeed made their way through a semi-aquatic evolution. This was a time when much of the land mass became covered with brackish water. Humankind evolved very rapidly from a knuckle-walking ape *(ramipithicus)* to the upright walking hairless early humans *(austrolapithicus),* who were contemporaries of the renowned Lucy. We evolved quite rapidly in a short time, as far as mutations go. The time passed in these huge inland bodies of water was spent fleeing predators and looking for food; we began to eat some shellfish and other easily gathered sea life. We lost body hair and adopted the more practical layer of subcutaneous fat like other mammals—dolphins and whales—that made the journey from land back into the sea. Like them, we copulate face-to-face, unusual in the animal kingdom. Our voices became developed since sound is crucial to underwater communication; our soft palate developed to become the precision tool it is today, giving us the range of vocal sounds we enjoy and need for modern survival.[22]

In times of great change the Earth's creatures have adapted to fit in with the environment. Most people are aware that we have a cell-mediated immunity, though may be surprised to learn that we also have a chemical/bioelectric-mediated immunity as well.

About 400 million years ago antibodies, as we know them, and three other immune proteins, appeared. Before this point chemical/bioelectrical-mediated immunity is mostly what protected and nourished the cells. We have elements like lipoic acid within us that protect and nourish our DNA. These colloids are smaller than 3-gigahertz wavelengths of light and can be found in fresh seeds and nuts. Let's look at the profile of a person with AIDS who does not have the immune cells in the blood that mediate immunity. If this person were to live in a healthy way with proper LifeFood hygiene, their chemical/bioelectrical-mediated immunity would begin to work for them again. Doctors are often puzzled as to how it is possible for an AIDS patient to have good health while simultaneously having a low level of T-cells and other indications of cell-mediated immunity. LifeFood cleans up dirty blood and gets busy safely emptying toxic organs. LifeFood offers the body superb building materials to make blood slippery and loosen and cart away debris.

The elements of our body are either composed of material colloids from LifeFood that possess a high resonance or of material colloids from denatured foods that have a lower vibration. Cooked starch, cooked protein, and cooked fats can have caused the ground base substance of our blood to be less discreet, meaning that fat forms on the body, especially during certain times in the lifecycle.

Uric acid and other broken down byproducts of proteins cause a dissolving of spores (viruses). Excessive drinking of non-alkaline beverages and acidic water can dilute uric acid. During fasting the body cleanses and the process of autolysis begins. This is when the aggregate colloids of the protein of cells being lysed (cleansed) are dissolved. Virus spores can form from these assembled colloids if they are not cleansed away through fasting and LifeFood in the diet.

Biologists have mistaken these virus spores as the core cause of a disease; however, this is only a partial truth. The resonance of these life colloids can cause a lysing of similar body structures. Which arrive directly from the breakdown of materials in our body.

David and I have looked at so many people's blood over the years, their living blood, their blood profile, and oxidative stress test on the blood. We have had the opportunity to witness the most dramatic recoveries and have seen time and time again a person completely change their blood profile in a relatively short period of time.

It's good to remind yourself that what is considered science is simply a collective agreement. Some may argue that new observations are entirely unscientific. What is accepted science today is different than agreed upon truths of the past—yesteryear's science. We present the information here in simplistic terms, and also in terms that need simplifying, because we are using a language that employs nuances of this present age. Before something becomes agreed upon collectively it may have been considered unscientific. This is just a reminder as you read though this work that you will need to make your own conclusions and observations of the terrain we offer.

Every day we get to witness miracles in our work. It's a thrill to observe a person clean up their blood. We witness people transform high blood pressure, liver, kidney, and heart challenges, and a whole host of other health conditions, to regain very good vitality in a matter of weeks.

In nature, you mostly see healthy animals, birds, and fish even though the wild is teaming with bacteria, spores, mold, and fungus—many of them carcinogens and pathogens. These toxins are kept at bay because of the animals' robust immune systems. The healthy first three stages of the lifecycle, beginning with colloids of life, or somatids, indicate a healthy immune system (growing phase); however, if the animal were to lose that vitality then the chief undertakers of nature transmutate into the world of mold, fungus, yeast, parasites (dying phase). All things in nature could be evaluated as either in their growing phase or their dying phase. This is observable everywhere around us as we watch the forest floor swallow up an enormous fallen tree, breaking it down into nothing over time. Take a quick look into the compost pile teeming with life. Even urine, which happens to be among the most sterile fluids of the body, will give rise to bacteria and ferments given time and the proper conditions.

We are highly electrical beings. So much so that energy radiating off a healthy person's fingertips can disassemble yeast. We become almost super-human with our robust immune systems. Staphylococcal food poisoning and other enterotoxins are stopped dead in their tracks by friendly ferments in the tummy. Your terrain is everything. Pleomorphic organisms can arise out of the terrain of the body without unnecessary vaccinations or other inoculations!

Most vaccination is purely useless and can be terribly damaging. It mistakes tolerance for immunity. The thinking person who examines vaccination and has a look at the clinical trials and the epidemiological trends of a disease will always conclude that a disease was on the decline when a vaccine was introduced. When Jonas Salk ran clinical trials for his polio vaccine no one in the placebo group contracted polio; however, 200 people he vaccinated ended up exhibiting symptoms of the disease. Polio, like all disease epidemics, was eradicated through the community pulling together to improve hygiene, improve nutrition, increase public awareness, and boost morale. Polio is passed from one person to the next by the process known as fecal/oral contact—a hygiene issue. It's interesting to note that each disease has an emotional component to it. Polio, for instance, arose out of the Depression, a time when the country was financially "crippled." This analogy was repeated over and over in the media and on the lips of the people who felt betrayed, a sense of frustrating helpless that hung like a cloud over America during the late 1930s. Polio is a disease that cripples children, the most psychic and resonant part of the community. It showed a remarkable decline once the country was "back on its feet" again. These were also the "Dirty Thirties," where most all the crops were lost to plague-like swarms of locusts and the topsoil blew across the land and into the sea. America had to completely rebuild its agricultural system, causing the food scarcity and poor quality of food because of the loss of minerals in the soil during these windstorms. Again, hygiene, proper nutrition, education, and a raised morale are the eradicators of disease. A boosted immune system is always the best guard against disease.

Another story that relates to boosted immunity is one of a nurse who traveled through poor southern communities after the smallpox plague had ravished America from 1775 to 1782. The nurse wrote in her diary that she came upon a little shack of a house where smallpox had killed the entire family with the exception of the littlest girl who was about seven years old. The nurse interviewed the child to try to determine how she had survived while the others had perished. The child told her that they were brutally poor and had lived on potatoes only. Her mother would peel them and boil them for the family to eat at dinner. It was the little girl's job to bring the potato peelings out back to the compost pile, and she was in the habit of eating most of the raw peelings along the way. This seemed to be the only habitual difference between her and the rest of the family. Was it the enzymes in the peelings that saved her? Smallpox is extremely virulent; smallpox scabs that sat on a researcher's shelf for thirteen years still had live, infective virus! What is it that gave this little girl the immunity edge? How could she live among this virulent virus and be seemingly unaffected?

Immunity

Spores, double spores, and viruses arise out of the simple colloidal substrate of the body depending upon the terrain. Even microbe-crazed Louis Pasteur, from whom we get pasteurization, said upon his deathbed, "The microbe is nothing, the terrain everything." It's almost unheard of for wild animals to have cancer. In sharks it is very rare, though less rare as the oceans become more polluted. In the last one hundred years almost one-third of all known life has disappeared from the earth. There has been a rise of anaerobic life forms. We have had a steady drop in the gauss nerve force. We have less oxygen and carbon dioxide. We have a gross imbalance of positive ions in cities, where the ratio can be as disparate as 600 positive ions to 1 negative ion. (Near a waterfall in nature that ratio is 1,000 positive ions to 1,150 negative ions.) There is a great historical rhythm to Earth changes, and all these things fluctuate with the seasonal equinoxes.

Our evolutionary path branched away from sharks many millions of years ago. Yet, sharks mark a divide when it comes to the world of immunity. Until recently it was assumed that sharks lacked the pivotal immune proteins that mammals have, and yet, regardless of this, they had excellent immunity. It has been found that they instead have elements within them that help them dissolve protein colloids.

The base ground substance of our blood and plasma has a variety of ways of keeping clean. It's interesting to note that those creatures that evolved earlier than sharks had no antibodies, nor other pivotal proteins that humans and other vertebrate possess today. Health depends on maintaining the proper internal and external hygiene. This is what is pivotal in living a vital life. Our ancient chemical/bioelectrical-mediated immunity, along with four proteins (antibodies, T-Cell Receptors, MHC, and RAG proteins), which are present in sharks as well as vertebrate life forms (from bony fish to mammals), keep our internal terrain hygienic and well ordered. This ancient immunity involves so few proteins it is primarily accomplished through a chemical mediated effect.

Sea urchins, insects, sponges, and other such life forms lack antibodies and T-cells. Yet, within these life forms, and in the base ground substance of vertebrate blood plasma, there are enormous amounts of immune protectors and cell modulators that enhance cell respiration and restoration. Sharks produce squalamine, a substance that dissolves spores and foreign protein.

Other more primitive life forms have cells that produce chemicals such as cytokines and cells that wander and engulf bacteria, helping to maintain the life forms' proper structure of colloids and cells in their bodies. There are other chemicals that lyse/dissolve dysbiotic life forms and primitive life forms that have natural antibiotics (pacifarins). The liver of a healthy person provides an array of needed nutrients. Health restoration may require a fresh source of colloids that comes in from LifeFood. Exogenous enzymes are needed to rebuild organs and other body systems, involving a streamlined coordination between the body systems.

Autoimmune Challenges Explained

Most important in this base ground substance we have been reviewing are the finer lipoproteins, smaller than a wavelength of light that nourishes and protects the DNA of our cells from AIDS and other immune-challenged conditions. As we stated before, sea urchins and sponges lack antibodies and T-cells. Much of the immunity that exists for them at this primitive level also exists within us, and it's clear that proper nutrition and a healthy lifestyle and environment affect the proper formation and integrity of this base ground substance.

Many things can challenge our vitality. Antibodies and immune cells can attack the very substance of our body tissue, mistaking them as foreign proteins. The body can form antibodies from consuming pasteurized milk from cows. Those antibodies can mistake the islets of Langerhans in the pancreas for a foreign protein because the heat-processed milk is an oligopeptide and the islets of Langerhans have similar proteins. Antibodies and other pivotal immune proteins like T-cell receptors, MHC proteins, and RAG proteins can form in the ground substance to attack disassembled (lysed) myelin sheathing (brain/spinal cord) as a result of low colloidal integrity of the fat/lipid-like materials that the myelin sheathing is composed of. If the myelin sheathing is composed of colloids of disassembled heat-processed fat (rancid fat), a person can develop antibodies to the debris in their own colon. Additionally, a person with these conditions can experience adhesions of fibrin and globulin, and tars and resins mixed with yeast cells and other mucus matter.

Cooked, denatured, poorly digested food in a body full of mycotoxins creates poor blood serum integrity. A person who boasts of not having a cleansing reaction—"never been sick a day in my life"—can actually stave off a major illness by having an acute cleansing reaction. All things in this world have a positive intention, even illness, or what we call a cleansing reaction or a need for a cleansing reaction. Illness causes a person to examine their hygiene, diet, lifestyle, and friendships; it slows you down so you have time to contemplate things. By honoring these factors in a good way one can bypass larger illnesses later in life.

Using live blood cell analysis microscopes, David and I have seen the full range of blood profiles—from perky well-formed blood to the opposite end of the scale where the blood is much like a trash heap. Many things we've discussed here can alter plasma terrain and blood profiles. It's easy to see a client's plasma, and other indices in their blood profile, respond dramatically to diet and lifestyle changes, turning around the mayhem that eu-stress from physical exertion and other stress substances have caused.

The body produces cortico-steroids that, unless properly neutralized by Vitamin B3, can cause havoc to the thymus gland, which is located by the center of chest. Other conditions, like absorbing powerful solvents, and parasites in the body, further aggravate this important gland. A person can develop antibodies from auto-inoculations of germs mixed with keratin containing skin cells (say from biting the fingernails) that mistakenly attack and disassemble colloids of the thymus gland because the thymus and the fingernails have many similar properties. It's crucial here to debulk the body and disassemble (lyse) the fat because many poisons cause free-radical damage unless a person is properly protected by a vital blood profile rich in spare electrons. As one cleanses the fat away, fat-soluble toxins are released.

The albumin to globulin ratio in a healthy person is about 2 to 0. Lifestyle and environmental toxins, as well as nu-toxins, can cause the production of too many blood cells than should be in a healthy body. Red, along with extra white blood cells, can be excessively produced. All these changes are adjustments the body makes to adapt itself to its environment, even if apparently less vital systems have to be sacrificed to maintain overall homeostasis.

Proper colloidal protein integrity of blood has to be in its isotonic state. This is achieved due to the fineness of particles and the electrically negative charge that each particle emits, helping to keep everything flowing. Otherwise, the terrain will allow crystallization of the colloids. The body can manage approximately seventy-five grams of protein in the blood at any given period of time and 75 percent of this should be albumin/high-density lipoproteins.

Because people eat mucus-forming foods, primarily starches, cleansing the cells of the body may require extra white blood cell production for digestion to occur. It will require the production of more antibodies, which is an acquired immunity that recognizes antigens and helps the body distinguish what is *self* and what is *other than self* (toxin or other debris). Maintaining proper internal hygiene requires having excellent physical and biochemical protective mechanisms factors. Some of these factors include the skin, digestive juices, inflammatory and healing responses, and cells that disassemble bacteria and tumors. All of these factors are specific morphology responses effected to ensure the maintenance of cell homeostasis.

The body's endocrine system provides a variety of information substances that are the key to youth. Nature has provided life forms with protective substrates like DHEA.[23] Cell cultures perform remarkably, even totally managing cytotoxic carcinogens like aflotoxin (a fungus in foods like peanuts, corn, cashews, and packaged bread). DHEA blocks sugars that are being turned into fats and nucleic acids and RNA and DNA. G6PD, the enzyme DHEA blocks in this process of sugar to fat, also causes cell abnormalities and appears to be involved as a causative factor in neoplastic[24] cells. There is more protein in our blood than any other substance, and their vast range and chemical composition causes an enormous variety. These proteins mainly come from liver cells and Kupffer cells within the endothelialsystem.[25]

Serum protein that provide nutrients to the brain, such as the very fine HDLs, may not be prevalent enough in a body where its forces have been crowded out by blood and plasma elements because of a need to clear and clean debris. Hygiene involves proper eating habits, otherwise the body will intervene in order to cleanse. And while it may have been possible that there was a seeming robustness prior to this point, the moment the body decides to cleanse, a person's blood profile changes radically. Some people will have relatively easy cleansing reactions, and others may really be put through the ringer to clear deep stubborn material from the deep folds of the body. To heal you may have to be strong enough to initiate you own cleansing process.

Sponges, sea urchins, and insects are completely without antibodies and T-cells, yet they are living evidence of a primitive immune protection that helps them—and other more advanced species—maintain environmental cell homeostasis. Denatured, heat-processed proteins can rob protein-splitting enzymes from a person's body and cause red blood cells to clump rather than flow discreetly. Particles of undigested protein from cooked food can caused nu-toxins and bacteria to arise from within. Antibodies, our T-cells, and NK lymphocyte cells are part of our acquired immune system. Antibodies, produced by B-cells in our blood plasma, are designed to recognize foreign proteins (antigens).

Antibodies specifically bind to antigens, tagging this debris in order for it to be removed or its structure disassembled. Antigens on the outside of bacteria and other antigens that have arisen can be tagged by antibodies so that debris can be disassembled and cleared by immune cells. Our immune system has novel ways of dealing with antigens and foreign growths and can even cause them to be chemically induced to explode as debris is identified and eliminated.

In all immune challenges and congenital conditions where one is without cell-mediated immunity we see how challenging it is to get along without antibodies and immune cells. We have evolved more than 100 million distinct antibodies that can bind to antigens to help us intercept a fantastic array of microbial dysbiotic elements. The body must maintain proper acid/alkaline balance for protein synthesis to occur. All enzymes have a pH range that they operate within, and good immunity requires having protein-splitting enzymes to break immune complexes down and having an intelligent and clear system where B-cells are educated to be aware of what antibodies to produce. This is only a small part of the picture.

T-cells, another part of our immune system, recognize antigens by means of proteins in their cell membranes called T-cell receptors. However, antibodies do not need MHCs,[26] a class of immune proteins that T-cell receptors require. T-cells require MHCs in order to bind to foreign protein in the body.

LifeFood and its cache of enzymes are needed by cells during healing to cut and paste genes so that information substances can arise that allow body homeostasis to be maintained. Antioxidants turn genes on and off; this process is activated from outside the cell. Enzymes are protein-derived material with a biotic life force that causes colloidal substances to be assembled or disassembled through resonance. DNA enzyme chopping of RAG protein in more evolved life forms is the same as it is for simple life forms like bacteria. Information substances often perform their work in the cell as they do in every other location in the body.

Enzymes are a necessary nutrient that the body needs. The body was designed for food to be digested and moved through the alimentary canal within about twelve hours. The colon is the body's sewer system. If someone eats three times during the day then they should defecate three times the following day. A sluggish colon and a fatty liver can cause the body to poorly maintain its oxidative metabolism.

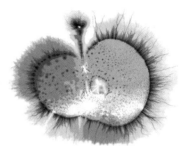

CHAPTER 4

The Procession of the Equinoxes

We are all familiar with the fact that our moon evolves around the Earth, and that Earth evolves around the sun, as all planets within our solar system do. Our solar system is also evolving around an enormous central sun called Alcyone that lies deep within the Pleiades star cluster toward the center of our galaxy. This revolution around Alcyone is called the *procession of the equinoxes*. It refers to the 26,000 years it takes for our solar system to make the journey—a long slow ellipse—once around Alcyone. Every 26,000 years, or to be more accurate 25,920 years, Earth has a birthday. There are dramatic influences that we go through during each phase of this evolution. It affects Earth changes like ice ages, pole shifts, and rapid evolution, or the digressing evolution of consciousness for the people; most remarkably our memory patterns, rates of cultural development, and technological advancement.

There are dramatic seasons to the procession of the equinoxes that directly affect us. During the 25,920-year procession there are times when we are much closer to the center of our galaxy and times when we are very, very far away from it. When we are heading toward the center we can observe states of rapid evolution and stunning leaps in technology in our history. When we turn the ellipse and head away from the center we forget all of our advancements and revert back to a very simple type of living. Ancient writings, primarily from India,

China, Egypt, and Iraq, document the procession of the equinoxes in great detail, though we have only "remembered" it again recently, as we enter the awakening time. The ancient Incan and Mayan peoples knew about the procession. The ancient Mayan calendar is one of the most accurate and hasn't been improved upon since. Our modern calendar is childish when compared to the sophistication and refinement of the Mayan calendar with its progressive understanding of the moving celestial bodies and their influence upon Earth and its people. It's obvious that these things were once known and then forgotten.

After the decline of the majestic civilizations of Egypt and ancient Sumer (today's Iraq), which enjoyed evolved government, written language, fabulous art, beautiful fine woven garments, and dramatic architecture, like the pyramids and sphinx in Egypt or the temples at Angkor Wat in Cambodia. These structures demonstrate a refined understanding of astronomy, and these cultures' well-ordered cities boasted highly efficient irrigation systems and cultivated agriculture. We have witnessed a dramatic fall from consciousness, where the people seem to have forgotten all of these things and have reverted back to gathering wild plants and hunting wild animals, and now have even severely digressed in areas of agriculture, written language, industry, art, and government.

Today we would be hard-pressed to reconstruct the Great Pyramid of Giza with the quarrying, movement, and placement of some 2 million stones—especially when you consider its stunningly accurate use of sacred geometry dimensions, including perfect Fibonacci and golden mean spirals. Try to fathom the ancient Egyptians' accuracy and understanding of the cosmos: If you start at the great pyramid and draw a line straight through the earth to its opposite point, measuring the circumference, and then take each point of the circumference and run them straight up to the center of the moon, and then run a line from the center of the moon to the exact center of the earth, it ends up being the precise proportions of the great pyramid (51 degrees, 51 minutes, 24 seconds)! Hardly the typical calculations included in today's construction projects, to say the least.

The great pyramid, and to an even greater degree the sphinx, are in fact much older than currently dated. This mis-dating of ancient artifacts is, for the most part, due to the fact that Moslems and Christians are held to follow what is commonly believed is the date of creation/ genesis in the Bible and Koran, which is generally put at 6,000 years ago (or 4,000 B.C.). Nearly all Egyptologists are Moslems who tend to have a particularly low tolerance for documentation that might discount this dating,[27] and so this falsification has been promoted for many Egyptian relics, and perhaps influences much of the information that we receive from sources bound to religious doctrines. Religious doctrine governs much of science (science: that which is generally agreed upon by a majority); it was only 1984 that the Vatican reversed its official proclamation that the Earth was at the center of our solar system, though for years it has been known that the sun is. Poor Galileo Galilei, in 1633, a man ahead of his time, was forced to lie to the court about his belief in Copernicus's theory—that the sun is central to our solar system. Regardless, he was arrested and publicly humiliated for a belief he publicly denounced, eventually leading to his death. The Roman Catholic reversal came more than a century after it was widely known that the sun was central to the solar system. Yet, embarrassment prevented the church from changing its stance on the issue. Over the years scientists and other religious intellectuals must have felt some angst at revealing their observations of nature if it would contradict official religious doctrine. Humans tend to regard their own personal belief systems to such a high esteem that many wars have been fought over defending personal and community principles.

Getting back to the procession of the equinoxes, for 13,000 years[28] our solar system was moving on its elliptical path away from the center of our galaxy, a time when consciousness had fallen asleep; Over the past 900 years we have rounded the turn and set on a course back toward the center of the universe to where we are today, at the awakening part of our journey.

We have been on the awakening part of this cycle for some time now; some say our official "Awakening" began on January 23, 1997, when a unique astrological formation appeared in the celestial heavens. Virtually all of the celestial bodies aligned in a sacred geometry shape of two inverted pyramids to form a perfect star tetrahedron—the Earth taking an important position in this configuration that occurred around the sun.

We are presently at a period during the procession of the equinoxes when the poles of the Earth shift. Pole shifts usually occur about 900 year after turning back from either end of the oblong ends of the ellipse. Pole shifts tend to create Earth changes and major changes in consciousness, which are magnetically oriented, much in the same way our memory records things and how most recordings today are magnetically oriented—from CDs, to audio tapes, to video tapes. Earth's nerve force, measured in gauss, has progressively ebbed now to its lowest point in recorded history.

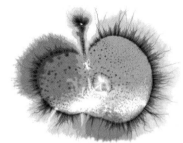

CHAPTER 5

Feeding the Light Body

Mineral Colloids and Manna from Heaven Awaken the Light Body

There is a sweet spot in our being that is the sum of two waves coming together and completely canceling each other out. Yet, even two of exactly the same waves are less than exactly the same in nature, so what's left over after the two waves have canceled each other out is a type of resonance. Two waves equal and opposite implode and leave behind a zero-point residuum wave. Zero point and its residuum wave are the energy that create or annihilate electrons. Wisdom of the ancient ones refers to this energy that rises from zero-point resonance as lunar pingala nadi and white spiral energy. Zero-point residuum wave energetics and superconduction cause us to have an aura, called the Meisner effect.

Zero point is when two oppositely projected polarized particles implode and unite into one through centripetal compression. The residuum wave that comes about from this is what fuels our light body. We have a physical body and a light body. For growth and proper cell respiration to occur, our physical and light bodies require nourishment, which LifeFood generously supplies.

Inner light, produced by zero-point residuum wave energetics, causes us to possess a bioenergetic field that is a polar complete energy produced by a single frequency of light coming from superconduction.

The most amazing thing about colloids of monatomic[29] elements is the property of superconduction they give us, even at room temperature. Amazingly, without being connected physically, energy flows from one superconductor to the other, as long as there is similar resonance between the two.

Blood carries the highest vibrational frequency (in the 80 kHz range) in the body along with the pineal gland. In health, the pineal gland cycles around 70 to 75 kHz. To enhance blood and pineal gland functioning, drink tea prepared from herbal colloid made from the herb chamaebatiaria nelleae (chamae). This herb is unique in that it retains its zeta potential regardless of temperature.

Amazing properties are drawn through the roots of this shrub from the soil where it grows. Drinking chamae tea releases its amazing cache of light-bearing phytochemicals that feed our light body. Chamae has a resonant frequency of 88 kHz. This is quite high for a living organism! And especially high for something which is seemingly less than "living."

Monatomic elements provide us with energy to interface with cells. Through the resonance from these elements, light floods into places where mutant DNA is corrected. The brain typically operates at 10 percent of its capacity. Yet, with LifeFood and this understanding of colloidal biology you can become more alive and conscious. This work teaches you how to feed your light body.

The term *manna of the Gods* refers to the process of tapping into free-energy and producing electrons from zero-point residuum wave energetics. In the sweet (alkalinity) extracellular fluid in our bodies, tachyons[30] are condensed into electrons. Alkaline energetics emits a friction grid that is continuously imploding the ethos. This is where electrons spontaneously materialize.

Through our way of living, we can feed our light body in a manner that grows this light until it is exceeding the body, until finally your body is emitting quite a lot of light. We've all met people that appear to glow. Certain emotions, like new love, can charge up the light body so that people cast off a soft yellow light for a period of time. Having spare electrons allows this glow to be a more permanent condition. Coal evolves through to its endpoint as a diamond. Rubies evolve from aluminum. The highly evolved Kung Fu master sends her opponents flying without ever delivering a physical blow; she simply throws her chi impeccably, evidence of a superbly refined light body and the ability to manipulate that energy.

Learning how to feed your light body is the very substance of this work. Colloidal biology is the manna that has assisted many enlightened people since the dawn of time to properly feed the light body. An evolved state comes from this understanding, which is complete joy and ecstasy. It is our birthright to be psychic, telepathic, and empathic. These are God-given gifts, though they are rarely developed and appreciated in modern society. Regardless, they are part of who we are; they are tools, like all cognitive skills, that become sharpened with practice and by increasing our intake of LifeFood and colloidal minerals. The physical senses sharpen and the sense of smell becomes quite developed as the dried-on mucus we've accumulated over the years is dissolved through LifeFood. That alone would be fine, but the sense organs evolve by taking on the properties of the higher quality materials the body is absorbing and so their function improves. The nerve-to-brain impulses from sense organs also become sharper, with a better electrical rhythm, with better synapse-firing in the brain, and so the entire sensory system, from stimulation to brain reconnection and response, is measurably improved.

One more interesting note is that LifeFood, because of its purity and electrical properties, contains the wisdom of nature. All food has an electrical field; even dead food has a very low amplitude of electricity. Within this electric field is contained the story of the food, in the same way your energetic field contains the story of your body, something a psychic person can read from the vibes you emit. The field cast from LifeFood is more or less directly from the seed to the field, from the soil, the water, the sun, the handpicking, and perhaps the journey in a truck to the market. In contrast, take a box of dried children's cereal, like Coco Puffs, or Apple Jacks, where, sure, somewhere in its history is contained the experience of the wheat field; but it is then harvested in enormous trucks called wheat thrashers, stored in a silo for many years, put through massive, loud grinding machines to make flour, stored again, shipped in trucks, and dumped into huge mixing machines with tons of sugar, lots of artificial flavor and color, and other things like pharmaceutical-grade vitamins to make up for the fact that it contains not an ounce of nutrition. Now, the vitamins, flavoring, and coloring all came from chemical labs and have long histories, and their energy fields are imprinted with those histories.

You can see where we're going here. If it is true that the electromagnetic field around food contains its story, then the box of cereal has a long, complicated story while LifeFood has a simple story that is wise beyond imagination. We come alive with the great mystery of being when we eat food that is alive and wise in its own right.

So much of the food people eat today has been processed out of this inherent intelligence. Food that is "dumbed down" has obvious pitfalls. It's interesting to observe the faces of people who regularly eat the impersonal processed food from fast food restaurants. Do they look alive with the spirit of nature? A young brave able to race across the land if need be? Or, do they look slowed down from the processed denatured food with its many corporate imprints? Yes, many corporate hands have touched this food, leaving it very little intelligence. Money was made along the way—for the fast food packagers; for the plastic and paper package itself; and for the host of chemicals required to get it to the counter. From the torrent of pesticides, herbicides, and fungicides sprayed on the crops to the antibiotics, hormones, and steroids in the feed of the factory-farmed animals, large corporate hands pocket cash all along the way. Mostly it is chemical-makers that are getting filthy rich while everybody else gets little. So, LifeFood has quite a large political implication; it takes that flow of money and channels it directly back to the farmer and the care of the soil.

Monatomic Elements Light Us Up through Resonance

Colloidal minerals give us the ability to be masts for cosmic energy. Colloidal silica, the mineral that gives our skin "snap" and cleans up our blood, gives off a frequency when it is electrically stimulated, which is the predominant frequency the moon gives off! Cognitive and emotional functioning is enhanced by this frequency. Silica emits a hertz frequency of 786,482 Hz. This is a harmonic frequency for the body that causes electrical conductivity throughout the connective tissue and is fundamental in the maintenance of good health and the promotion of a long life. Healthy cells are also aglow with colloids of elements that are in an atomic high-spin state. Monatomic rhodium and iridium and ten other monatomic elements are very important light body elements.

Let's take a look at the monatomic world of the invisible, going all the way inside of our bodies to imagine the nucleus of an atom. It's surprising to find that some of the monatomic elements have nuclei that are oddball shapes, like footballs or bananas. Atomic nuclei are measured in units called firmes.[31] A small nucleus may only be a few firmes wide. The most remarkable thing you may notice is how vast the distance is between the nucleus and its orbiting electron cloud. The electron cloud around the nucleus is very far away—at a distance of as much as one thousand firmes!

We feel the moon is far away from the Earth, yet, relatively speaking it's quite close in comparison to electrons that are so far away from their nucleus. Packed in the nucleus that is three to four firmes wide and ten firmes long are the neuclons, mostly protons or neutrons, and the mass of the atom with its positive charge. The enormous mass of the nucleus of the atom comes from the nucleons, while the protons in the nucleus carry a positive charge.

Nuclei of atoms owe their structure to two unique interacting energies. There is a strong nuclear force holding the protons together, as well as a weak electromagnetic force repelling the protons from each other. The strong force acts over a short distance, within ten firmes, whereas the weaker coulomb force acts over a longer range.

All biological systems possess enzymes that cause larger elements to be divided and sectioned at the level of protons through harmonics. Enzymes biologically transmutate one element into another by simply combining or subtracting protons and electrons. The first twenty elements of the elementary chart especially take part in this process.

Elements that have nuclei where its protons are ten firmes or more apart can be easily undone. When this happens, time-forward and time-reverse electrons become paired and coexist as light. As a particle, the electron ceases to exist and it too becomes light. As this is happening, monatomic elements possess extraordinary properties.

Healthy body cells, as well as symbiotic organisms like primitive spores or cells (life colloids), have monatomic atoms that cause the life form to possess superconductivity. LifeFood's like fresh grapes and fresh aloe vera possess monatomic elements that feed your light body. Monatomic elements are high-spin atoms. Other high-spin atoms come from silver, platinum, nickel, copper, cobalt, mercury, palladium, osmium, and ruthenium.

Normal atoms have an energy field around their nucleus that typically screens the inner electrons to the atom in an orderly protected manner. It is typically the electrons on the outside that lend themselves for chemical bonding (valence electrons). However, elements in a high-spin state, where time-forward and time-reverse electrons implode together creating superconduction, have their fields especially expanded. These expanded fields help screen and protect and put order to all electrons, even those electrons on the very outer perimeter.

Atoms with electrons under this unique screening potential cause time-forward and time-reverse electrons to pair and harmonize and to become light. These particles of matter (electrons) become light! Various elementary particles that are in a monatomic state (light-bearing) as a colloid have time-reversed electrons that act like positrons (the energy originating in the nucleus).

Emission spectroscopy, which measures electron absorption and emission, as well as other instruments that analyze regular elements, are calibrated to pick up energetics on a three-dimensional plane. Superconduction is occurring on another plane where matter has become light! Most of these instruments are not sufficiently calibrated to interact with this energetic matter, since high-spin atoms have extraordinary properties.

Football- or banana-shaped nuclei come apart easily. Mother nature has created monatomic elements in the belly of the Earth and spews rhodium and iridium out through her volcanic vents. Monatomic elements such as rhodium, iridium, and palladium are in a high-spin state and create a tremendous release of energy. There is an enormous increase in amperage of energy that is released. These monatomic elements give us a light body that feeds on electromagnetic resonance. In the past, people believed that it was amperage that fed our light bodies, but it is our light bodies that set our amperage.

Within the body there are precious minerals in their colloidal form, which in a high-spin state build us an enormous amount of energy, much in the same way a capacitor works. Our prophets and exalted ones have light flowing out of their bodies. Whenever any one of these monatomic elements goes into a high-spin state other elements respond and begin to possess similar properties, including superconduction at room temperature!

Mercury can be divided down to the point of a fine white powder. For 4,000 years the ancients passed alchemical secrets to initiates showing how one might arrive at this white powder from mercury (its monatomic state). To test this powder to see if it was ready for consumption, one would combust it with a flame, for when it was ready it would glow a magnificent gold.

From Mercury to Gold

More powerful than a million volts, a photon can come flying from out of nowhere and into the nucleus of an element like gold, and rather than produce a light-bearing element can instead cause the element to become more solid. A high-speed photon coming into the nucleus causes atom protons and several neutrons to be changed. A photon can alter its spin to become slower, thus having the tendency to gather (aggregate) with other colloids of the same type to form the metal diatomic gold.

Beautiful and precious, there are few elements more precious than gold in its solid state. But there is something—gold that has been split in half to a white powder state. It is more valued in this form because it owes its form to an atom in a high-speed monatomic state that is precious in its efforts to help feed our light body. This creates a state of superconduction. Gold split in half can become rhodium or ruthenium. Silver minus a few protons and electrons can become rhodium. Gold and mercury minus a few protons and electrons can become platinum, iridium, or osmium.

Brain and nerve tissue is made up of a surprising amount of rhodium and iridium (5 percent of its dry matter weight). Our physical body and light body are interdependent systems. Liquid light that is invisibly scintillating and flowing around the body causes DNA to function in an orderly way.

Carcinogens can be pinned to DNA that cause light to be greatly compromised. The energy field and aura can be diminished or very low in the affected area of the body. For example, a person with hepatitis will show an implosion in their energy field outside the liver area. The less light that flows, the more heat can built up. When light flows around a carcinogen and heat builds up, the DNA pattern can be altered. When this happens, DNA strands have received too much heat! You can imagine a fuse wire burning out. When we bring light-bearing elements into our body, correct resonance can reestablish itself and mutated genes are healed because this superconductive light lifts and clears carcinogens away from the DNA, causing the cell to revert back to its normal architecture and proper cell function.

Healing involves the synergistic combination of quite a cascade of energy along with matter of the universe. These precious light-bearing minerals, in their high-spin state, allow the vestibular mechanism to act as control central, as an endolymphatic gravitational inertia device. Embedded in the temporal lobes, regulating impulses on a number of levels, the vestibular mechanism regulates impulses sent through sensory motor nerve cells and also, surprisingly, via the insulation material that coats nerve cells in our bodies. This latter energy causes a readiness potential long before any nerve impulse is actually sent.

Superconductive energy is totally responsible for nerve and growth processes. Superconduction occurs because life colloids, both simple and complex, employ monatomic elements. The high-spin atoms result in a resonant coupled system (a lining up of particles). A harmonious, stable external electromagnetic field is very important for superconduction to occur in biological systems. Superconduction in biological systems occurs in fields below 8 to 10 gauss at room temperature. Life colloids detect weak magnetic fields as much as .1 to 5 gauss. This is a productive electromagnetic field within which organisms respond.

The bioenergetic gravity field emitted from your hand can levitate superconductive material from six inches away! A magnet would cause nothing to happen in this same instance. Superconductivity can flow in enormous amperage—in the hundreds of thousands of amps—in response to the tiniest bioelectromagnetic gravity field! Living bodies have the equivalent amperage, upwards of 200,000 amps per square foot without any voltage! Even though an enormous current is flowing, you are without a trickle or even a spark.

Rhodium and iridium from fresh aloe vera, grape juice, and other nutrient forms of colloidal monatomic elements (the tea made from chamae), help organize and keep our DNA functioning naturally. As far as many of the present instruments are concerned, as superconduction is happening and two equal and opposite waves cancel each other out;

our three-dimensional instruments cannot efficiently gauge high-spin atoms because the electron and the positron are in perfect harmonics. A residuum wave arising from this cancellation cannot be effectively measured. As two particles are imploding they leave a residuum vibration that is known as a planckian frequency.[32]

Overtone chanting, practiced by people in older cultures like Tibet or Aboriginal Australia, cause this planckian frequency to rise within us. This is timelessness in the universe. This is the interaction of zero-point energy at the center. As equal and opposite vibrations implode into each other they become null and void and nothing. The residuum frequency left behind is what interacts on the level of DNA.

This bioelectromagnetic zero point is within us, and within all life. It is what holds living matter together. It is singularity. This is where particles are born within us, out of a vacuum, each and every moment of the day. Electrons can appear and disappear. Within an electromagnetic zero point, these precious minerals, in their high-spin state, emit light resonance coupled as a low-energy coulomb wave to release tremendous amounts of an orderly type of energy. These precious elements of the Earth make life possible, and when we harness them we tap into free-energy. These precious minerals act like a gate releasing the nuclear energy contained within the nucleus of the very atoms that we are composed of and turning it into electromagnetic energy.

Gravity and Electricity Are Related

Electrogravitic force fields permeate the universe. They bend and influence the speed of light and create the colors of the rainbow. Yellow indicates new life, while a shift to red is indicative of disease. A pendulum takes a shorter time to swing through its arc when negatively charged (lighter) than when positively charged (heavier). Producing an inverse electromagnetic field neutralizes a gravitational force field. We are lighter while we have life force. This is our ability to convert tachyon energy. The enormously concentrated nuclei of atoms are actually smaller than presently calculated because of electrogravitic interaction.

This is the reason they are so sturdy and difficult to collapse.

Colloids resist the pull of gravity. Each one is like a planet in a miniature solar system. These minute mineral particles measure about 400,000th to 400,000,000th of an inch. If one cubic inch of life colloids were flattened onto a sheet one-colloid thick, it would cover one-and-a-half acres! Colloids of life can resist temperatures of 3,000 degrees and have survived exposures to nuclear radiation of up to 50,000 rems! Life colloids (bacteria) even live in water that cools the reactor core in nuclear power plants. In the future organisms will be used to biologically transmutate radioactive materials into inert materials like silver. Life exists even with this amount of radiation! They keep their form even through humans attempt to cut them with a diamond knife.

Cells Are Formed from Mineral Colloids

Organic structures are built out of colloids. Mineral colloids, depending upon the morphogenic energy field, assemble into primitive life forms. Life colloids are formed from mineral colloids. In fact, all organic and inorganic materials are formed from colloids. Colloids are the material (as life colloids) from which we get our shape. Given the right conditions, colloids of life (life colloids) aggregate together to form spores, whether these primitive forms of life exist in soil, plant, or animal. Aggregates of mineral colloids assemble as spores aggregate together to form double spores. Double spores metamorph by fusing together to create a body cell or bacterium.

The colloids that make up the cells of our body primarily arrive as colloids that incorporate into red blood cells. Many of the cells of our body came from colloids that were originally red blood cells. Some mitotic cell division does occur, of course. However, most cells in our body are assembled from colloids that were previously disassembled from red blood cells.

Disassembled colloids, depending upon the morphogenic field they find themselves in, go through a process of aggregation, fusion, specialization, and in some situations, they even reassemble to form a nucleated cell! Colloids that comprise red blood cells (erythrocytes), even though they are without a nucleus, pool their cache of colloids to become a monera,[33] out of which a nucleated cell or even a multi-nucleated cell can assemble.

The shape of the life colloid that is formed depends upon the morphogenic field that influences its expression. Like movement in water or some other medium that energetically produces standing wave forms, these standing wave forms influence the bonding angle of hydrogen and oxygen. They also play a role in how water molecules fit together in nature's various characteristic life forms, from snowflakes to butterflies.

Everything is a matter of timing. The importance of resonance is its ability to act in a precision manner to give things character. All life forms have their natural set of frequencies that they vibrate to. Giant icebergs are splintered because of the resonance caused by the gentle lapping of waves. Resonance can allow a lot of little pushes in the right direction that when combined can create great momentum and achieve spectacular results. Witnessing the effect of resonance is a matter of literally being in the right place and time.

Colloids that become incorporated as a body cell, spore, double spore, or bacterium can disassemble from whatever form they take on and then reassemble into a cell wall, deficient bacterium, or mold. Mold can transmutate itself into fungus, just like a caterpillar can transform into a butterfly, as a biological process. However, fungi can biologically transmutate itself back into its more primitive form as mold, bacteria, double spores, single spores, somatids, or body cells.

Space Dust, Life Colloids, Dinosaurs, and Blood

Space dust gathers to form colloids of life. Colloids of life, or somatids, are billions of years old. The ones that once made up the dinosaurs now thrive in you and me! Everything we are composed of can be found individually in nature. Every conceivable organic and inorganic substance is made of colloids. All living things are made up of and depend on colloids. Colloids of life assemble from the soil to form plant roots (much like the microcillia of yeasts), which eventually become colloidal nutrients, which ultimately go on to become the structure of the fruit and vegetables we eat.

The earth is 70 percent water and 30 percent colloids; likewise, the body is 70 percent water and 30 percent colloids. These colloids come in an enormous variety of sizes, shapes, ingredients, and constituents, including seawater, blood, and fresh vegetable juice.

Key Factors that Constitute a Colloidal System

Colloidal systems consist of dissimilar, insoluble ingredients that can coexist as solids (particles), liquids, and/or gases at different concentrations, so long as particles of a smaller size variation exist outside the size of the colloids. Otherwise, if the colloids reached a high concentration, they would attract each other and fall out of their solution (gravity). If the combined colloids of the Earth exceeded 30 percent, it would affect the Earth's orbit and in turn effect a reaction from the other planets in our solar system.

Water Moves Stone

The earth is made up of rocks, among other things. If a large granite rock is placed in water, it sinks. Yet, during an ice age, stone is ground into powder of minute colloids that are so small they suspend in water. Boulders have been known to be suspended within the energy vortices in the bottom of a waterfall tier and be lifted to the surface. Spawning fish use this energy to jump up waterfalls. Small mineral colloids become suspended in the same way, repelling each other.

Colloidal Minerals as Vital as Vitamins

Mineral colloids are what conduct electricity in our bodies. Minerals are essential to body function. Bone, skin, hair, enzyme function, and circulatory activity all require colloidal minerals.

Vital health requires a broad range of some ninety minerals per day! The average person on a denatured diet may have received only three or four minerals in a given day! Most people transmutate one element into another, biologically exchanging protons with the atoms' nuclei to assemble the desired element. Friendly bacteria assist us in our ability to absorb minerals. It's silly to think that one could receive needed minerals by licking the earth. We are not equipped to absorb minerals in that form.

Alchemy of life colloids (phytoplankton, microbes) and plants assemble colloids from the soil and combine with them to create an organic form that we can incorporate for ourselves. The blood's colloid-mineral integrity could be compromised to start with because of poor soil and food that is denatured from processing and preparation techniques. Combine these factors with increased challenges due to individual stresses and you will begin to realize that you have to actively monitor your blood profile. Supplements might be advised in this case.

Bioavailability of Minerals

To benefit from mineral supplementation, one must mimic nature's colloidal mineral-organic combination. Life colloids are an intermediary step between minerals and us. If you found a lump of iron or took chromium from someone's bumper bar and chewed it, those minerals would be indigestible and toxic. Minerals need to be naturally combined with carbon to make them organic rather than inorganic. They have to be small enough and have a negative charge to be absorbed by the body.

Chemistry has concerned itself with the inorganic, organic (containing carbon), and colloidal properties of solutions. Chemistry has mostly focused on electron interactions; however, life force involves a study of subatomic interactions. Substances produced by the liver and kidneys, like picolinic acid, naturally chelate with minerals because picolinic acid has many spare electrons. Most people on a cooked, denatured diet have been unable to naturally chelate minerals because cooked food has made them picolinic-acid deficient! These are people who stuff themselves, yet are starving at the cellular level.

The benefit of every mineral and nutrient can easily be enhanced or diminished, depending on what type of delivery is employed. Optimal colloidal mineral reserves can be restored through improved consumption habits. Cooking food may have caused available colloidal minerals to lose their anionic charge and become more cationic. Cells cannot efficiently absorb minerals from cooked food because the membranes of our cells are made up predominantly of hydrogen ions. Hydrogen tends to be positive and two positives repel one another; cationic minerals also have a positive charge.

Bioavailability can be less than optimal when minerals are not in colloidal form, or when poor levels of digestive enzymes and intestinal nutrient assimilation compromise the integrity of these systems. Bioavailability is the measure of a nutrient's ability to cross the cell membrane and be assimilated within our cells. Colloidal nutrition should become the buzzword in professional and lay circles alike. Enzymes disassemble colloids of a nutrient, increasing its surface area, thereby enormously maximizing its bioavailability.

Insoluble, permanently suspended colloids can be smaller than a wavelength of visible light. Because of this they can emit a negative electrical surface charge and become isotonic. Our body fluids are isotonic and predominantly consist of colloidal suspensions with a negative charge. The process of digestion must render a mineral nutrient into a colloidal form for maximum nutrient assimilation.

Blood cells can have poor flow because of indiscriminate positive electrical potentials. These can be introduced either by cationic nutoxins, like aluminum and cadmium, or by electromagnetic sources, such as video display terminals. Since positive and negative charges attract each other, cells will clump together, limiting oxygenation of the body.

A vortex created in the heart continuously creates a negative charge for these colloids. Blood vitality involves keeping the blood cells discreet, thereby increasing the individual cell's transport area. As long as the blood is clean of fats and excess undigested protein and starches, blood cells retain their invigorating negative electrical charge.

Blood colloidal electrolytes help keep blood cell membranes electrically negative. Mineral colloids act as co-factors along with vitamins, helping enzymes do their work (as everything is made up out of colloids). Nutrients like co-enzyme Q10 help to fuel each cell's super-rich energy compound known as Adenosine Triphosphate (ATP). Cells use ATP for 95 percent of their energy requirements.

Mineral colloids join to become simple "life colloids." Colloids coming from a biological system are imbued with energy that colloids coming from the solid granite rock lack. Primitive life like bacteria, mold, yeast, fungus, and lichens interact directly with inorganic minerals to form colloids of life.

Phytoplankton, algae, and plants deliver minerals to us in their most assimilative form, for colloids have been part of a complex biological system. Minerals coming in the form of colloids from these natural biological life forms are imbued with vital energetics that minerals simply chelated with amino acids, or colloids put together in a laboratory, may lack.

Colloids of life draw their energy (phosphorylation of ATP) from oxidation in the presence of oxygen. Life colloids in the presence of oxygen break ATP down to a friendly lactic acid. Unfriendly life colloids without the presence of oxygen would break sugar down into ATP through fermentation, producing extremely toxic waste byproducts like acetaldehyde, methane, and ethyl alcohol. These mycotoxins in turn make the body more acidic and nutrient elements become congealed and coagulated. These colloids will then lose their solubility as they crystallize and become more acidic.

Water and the Chemistry of Life

Water makes up the largest component of the body. Seventy to ninety percent of all organic matter is composed of water. All enzymatic-sustained reactions take place in a fluid medium. Water is even a product of cellular metabolism. Hydrogen and oxygen tend to be positive and negative, respectively. Water, being a superb solvent, has a positive and a negative pole and has the ability to form weak bonds, which allow them to disassemble and reassemble during physiological reactions.

The electron of the hydrogen atom, along with the eight electrons of oxygen, is the key to life as we know it. Hydrogen alone has a single proton and a single electron. Water is made of combining two hydrogen atoms with one oxygen atom that has eight protons in its nucleus and eight electrons circling its orbit. Hydrogen is therefore combined with oxygen to make water, or is split apart to make ions. Hydrogen tends to be easily ionized, a process that occurs simply by losing a single electron. Hydrogen also bonds with other elements, sharing its simple electron with an atom in need of an electron, like oxygen.

Atoms Gain or Lose Electrons

Reduced atoms are given electrons; conversely, oxidation is the process of removing electrons. As electrons are given, energy is stored in the reduced compound; where electrons are removed (oxidation), energy is liberated from an oxidized compound. As one substance is reduced, the other is oxidized. Electron exchange constitutes the mechanism of oxidation-reduction (redox) reactions. A base (alkaline, OH-) decreases hydrogen ions, while an acid increases hydrogen ions (H+).

Negative Ions Are Released in Nature

Negative ions are created when free electrons are released by radioactive carbon, rubidium, and potassium in the soil and plants. Free electrons are released by the absorption of ultraviolet light by organic and inorganic matter. Low energy electrons are accelerated to a higher energy by way of an atmospheric voltage gradient: from 300 volts/meter at sea level to 7,000 volts/meter at 8,000 feet.

High-energy electrons impact oxygen and water to form byproducts, mainly secondary electrons of lower energy. These electrons go on to impact with other molecules, causing the release of additional electrons. Some become so low in energy that they stick to the impacted atom, giving it a negative charge and making it a negative ion. Negative ions are integral in isotonic fluids, like blood. Their negative charges keep the cells discreet, allowing for greater oxygenation.

Is Oxygen a Good Thing?

Oxygen is elemental to survival. The body uses oxygen atoms to disinfect, disassembling spores, bacteria, and other waste products. Oxygen is relatively stable in the air, however, if more oxygen is absorbed than the body can handle it becomes unstable. It would then have a tendency to join with molecules of healthy cells as free radicals. This chemical activity is due to the atoms having unpaired electrons and shifted electron belts, causing the atoms to seek stability.

Ordinarily, 2 percent of the oxygen that we breathe becomes active. When we exercise, this can go up to about 20 percent. However, oxygen atoms with unpaired electrons are unstable and extremely reactive. DNA damage can occur when active oxygen atoms attach themselves to healthy cell membranes and body tissue. These atoms have high oxidation (electron-stealing) potential. Health challenges, however, can arise when an overabundance of free radicals affect healthy cells.

Active oxygen robs electrons from proteins, fats, carbohydrates, and collagen, resulting in an array of undesirable byproducts like indole, scatol, phenols, ammonia, histamines, and hydrogen sulfide. These tissue toxins enormously challenge liver function. Putrefying and fermented food in the digestive tracts is often the cause of disease in the body.

Indoles and phenols that are active and unmanageable are carcinogenic. Histamines contribute to atopic inflammation of the skin and respiratory cells of the bronchioles and lungs. White blood cell leukocytes (neutrophils) scavenge electrons from colloids that are in need of being disassembled and then use these spare electrons to reduce acids. Challenges arise when the body is unable to handle free radicals. Lymphocytes, however, use active oxygen, like hydrogen peroxide, to oxidize bacteria, mold, fungus, and yeasts. The Lymphocyte, a healthy life colloid of our immune system, sends out a pseudopod (tentacle) that injects hydrogen peroxide or ascorbic acid to rob electrons from the undertaker life colloids (mold, fungus, yeast).

Health involves coping with this type of oxidative oxygen. The body is protected by neutrophils (leucocytes) and preserved by the alkaline pH of body fluids. Free electrons are given to oxygen free radicals, thus neutralizing their oxidative potential.

Antioxidants keep a body young and are an important element in physical resiliency. Antioxidants like pycnogenols, bioflavanoids, Vitamins C and E, selenium, and beta-carotene are reducing agents. Elements that have an abundance of electrons, such as essential fatty acids, help oxygenate the body.

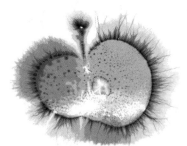

CHAPTER 6

Living Blood

Blood Condition Wants Life to Arise

Live blood cell analysis is fascinating. We can observe living, moving blood and the amazing things that go on in it. We can accelerate blood to pass completely through its lifecycle in a short time. Viewed through dark field microscopes, blood has life that can be seen as colloidal life forms assembling from the extracellular fluid. Colloids of life grow from red blood cells into the extracellular fluid. Colloids collect in a pool to form a mass of colloids called monera. Sometimes spicules appear between the red blood cells. This is where colloids have been expelled from red blood cells and mass into a hazy fog-like veil that starts to fade the microscope light.

Some virus spores found forming in the blood can survive heat of 300° Centigrade! They are very hearty. These simple colloidal life forms do not have nuclei. Colloids from mold, fungus, and yeast have an affinity for hybrid food. Red blood cells composed from these undertakers of life can ferment the colloid foodstuffs, causing the blood to develop acid-fast cell-wall deficient L-formed bacteria. The colloids are then expelled by the red blood cells, and may assemble into thrombocytes that can occlude blood vessels. With live blood cell analysis we see bacteria assemble before our eyes. It moves from the colloidal protein into the blood to assemble into three to five nuclei.

Understanding colloidal biology and the secrets of an alkaline body, you can learn to feed your light body and help educate others to feed theirs. Old science held to a process of passing blood through filters, and the proteins that were small enough to pass were called viruses. The old blind thought taught that viruses (spores) fixed forms as independent life forms. Today we understand spores to be byproducts of cell breakdown that assembles, disassembles, and reassembles into characteristic life forms. Depending upon the terrain, these protein-derived colloids can transform from one thing to another. They are malleable; if nature wants to express a healthy leukocyte, or a liver cell, or any cell for that matter, that's exactly what will be created. The marrow in our bones incorporates the very substance that comprises our whole being.

Colloidal simple life forms help keep our terrain intact! Colloidal biology can be used to disassemble bacteria, mold, fungus, and yeast back to their primitive forms by encouraging the pH of the terrain to transform to health. LifeFood colloidal nutrients are easily digested and assimilated and supply the body with the amazing array of materials to crowd out unfriendly bacteria, mold, fungus, and yeast and refresh the terrain of the body to a more youthful blood/lymph profile. On the other end of the scale, all processed/denatured food is acid-forming in the body so you find that when blood becomes extremely alkaline and the body tissue extremely acidic it is a ripe background for disease. That is the primary cause of so much premature death.

Healthy Blood Spins Right

A person may bring 1200 mg of ionic-bound calcium into the body from pasteurized sources like milk, cooked grains and greens, dolomite, or Tums antacid tablets; yet, only a little of that devitalized dead calcium is enlivened by intestinal flora. It is dead calcium that is often stored in occluding shelves and plaques that laminate the passageways and clog the sensitive glandular systems of the body. LifeFood is 80 percent alkaline and 20 percent acidic. Nutritive substrate colloids presented to the body in their natural organic covalent-bound form make them easy to absorb.

Healthy blood cells are abundant in number, are regular in size and type, and are flowing smoothly and discreetly. Blood is clean when it has healthy colloids of life. Blood that has a perfect pH of 7.3 keeps unhealthy pleomorphic development at bay. Healthy red blood cells have a slight spin to the right. Unhealthy blood is found in those suffering from electrochemical smog, one result of which is its bizarre left-spinning blood. The body's L-field is stimulated and strengthened through vital LifeFood and an active, playful, satisfying lifestyle.

Selected resonance results from a balanced lifestyle that causes the body's L-field[34] to regain a healthy frequency. This causes reticular magnetic energy emission that maintains the proper electron spin of the blood. The Earth is a huge magnet and everything, even the sea, is governed by magnetism and the pull of ions.

L-field harmony and emission come about as a result of having enough carbon inside our cells, about 7 percent. Carbon specifically emits a nerve force that enormously enhances our ability to deflect subnormal galvanometric energy. Relaxed and quiet, calm breathing helps induce and maintain this state. This type of breathing has an amazing effect on blood.

There are so many things one can do to improve their health. It's a fact that North Americans' favorite fruit and vegetable are the banana and the potato, respectively, both of which are hybrids that lack vital electrics and antioxidant nutrients. On any given day, the vast majority of people eat inferior food. Vitamin C in green beans, for instance, is reduced by 50 percent seven days after having been picked. There is the most amazing link between the Central Nervous System (CNS) and the level of geomagnetic activity (GMA). There is an increased flow of calcium ions through cell membranes as the body's L-field is in harmony. Cell membranes are liquid crystals that are temperature sensitive for energy flow.

The north (-) end of a magnet spins blood counterclockwise (left), decreasing hydrogen ions; whereas the south (+) end causes blood cells to spin clockwise (right), increasing hydrogen production. The control of the hydrogen ion is an important reaction that takes place in the body. Simply said, it is very good to have spare hydrogen ions available. It keeps us looking youthful.

Our Body Aura (L-Field)

The adrenals, pituitary, heart, thyroid, and gonads are involved in increasing hydrogen ions (acid), which inhibits the stomach, liver, pancreas, intestine, and bronchioles as hydrogen is increased. The sympathetic and parasympathetic systems work to speed things up or slow things down, respectively. As long as the body maintains its L-field, a person will have excellent immunity. Otherwise, harmless diploic and short-chain strains of streptococci mutate in an anaerobic (oxygen-deprived) condition. These pleomorphic organisms excrete virulent toxins that require the attention of the immune system, thus compromising the immune system.

The electrical currents in the body have strong magnetic fields. Magnetic energy flows through a neutral zone to join the its opposite polarity. Reticular magnetic energy (RE) flows through the body and is emitted out in a straight line. The body is a perfect conductor in the same way a crystal is. Certain plastics are effective barriers to this conduction. Reticular magnetic energy is one of three fundamental energies that cells use to communicate with each other without being physically connected. Reticular magnetic energy makes it easy for cells to propagate and is involved in information exchange between living cells. Reticular magnetic energy plays a major role in healing the body's terrain. L-fields are composed of body magnetic emanations. RE conducts through healthy tissue and selected tissue that needs to be recharged.

Synchronized hemisphere activity fed by heart/mind and heart/breath integration causes this magnetic flow to be flexed laterally out and away in a straight line from the body. This is RE energy. Life is influenced by environmental RE energy. We draw on RE energy from our environmental surroundings to maintain good health, as do the symbiotic organisms living within us.

Warm Alkaline Body, Inactivate Spores

Blood inhibitors influence the healthy expression of life colloids in living tissue along with healthy cells. Thus, blood and tissue pH is vital, as pleomorphic expression will occur in overly alkaline blood and/or acidic tissue. Cells lyse and break down into spores, like herpes, under conditions of cold and acidic tissue. Warm and alkaline tissue maintains vital tissue integrity.

Eruptive herpes blisters are a form of cell lysing, where cells are limited to certain available channels for mobilizing mineral reserves to maintain nerve and body tissue integration. Spores have a resonance that causes tissue to disassemble (lyse). The mucous membrane of the eyes, lungs, and bowels, where blood has maintains less than vital qualities, can allow pleomorphic expression beyond symbiotic life colloids. Body tissue that under a pH of 6.8 is acidic and cannot block neoplastic growth (cancer). A cool and acidic environment encourages cell lysing, while warm alkaline environments inactivate virus spores.

LifeFood produces an ideal tissue pH that completely allows tissue integrity to remain. You could say that resonance is maintained. The body naturally produces substances that dissolve viruses through resonance in the same way a vibrato singer hits a high C note, shattering crystal glass with the sound wave. Natural phytochemicals, like those in narcissus, persimmon bark, winter grape root, lomatian, and lemon balm, can be consumed to engage the body's vital biological response to neutralize and dissolve virus and mold spores. Herbs should be taken as fresh compounds. Two other herbs great for lysing foreign virus spores are horehound and yarrow. These herbs are long proven and written about; the Bible mentions wormwood— a wonderful antibiotic that has natural pacifarins.

Laser technology and ultraviolet light are now combined together in a microscope to illuminate that which has only been seen by clairvoyants until recently. Blood and other biological liquids have been observed to possess colloids of life endowed with movement that has a variable lifecycle of multiple forms. There is a diversity and evolved sequence appearance of these life colloids as they aggregate into spores, double spores, bacteria, mold, fungus, and yeast.

Trace minerals and organic substrates act as blood inhibitors to regulate the life colloids' lifecycle so that it does not exceed double its spore stage. These inhibitors allow primitive life colloids to live in saphritic relationship with us and produce substrates like growth hormone and help the body dissolve dysbiotic life forms through eco-sterilization. In universities that still use stained smears of dead blood analysis, the remains of pleomorphic organisms are called "artifacts" or "fibrin formations."

When alkaline buffers in tissue and nerve force are compromised, harmful mycobacterium evolve and then burst to release yeast-like forms at the fungal level. It evolves through *ascosporic* to *asci* and is distinguished in modern labs as small lymphocytes. Yet, asci grow and burst and liberate new life colloids to start the entire pleomorphic lifecycle again, if a good and healthy terrain allows it (alkaline blood/ acidic tissue). B-lymphocytes secrete antibodies that cause dysbiotic pleomorphic organisms (unhealthy bacteria) to lose their cell walls.

Food, Mood, and Surroundings Build Blood

Photons of light have a natural interaction with living matter, measurable at a cull level. Biology is extremely sensitive to extremely low frequency (ELF) electromagnetic waves. All microorganisms react to a particular frequency. We have seen spores change into bacteria and bacteria change back into spores! Dysbiotic microscopic life forms can be targeted and dissolved through ultrasonic resonance.

After a meal of denatured foodstuffs filled with colloids close to assembling into mold, fungus, and yeast, a person's blood can resemble that of a person with cancer! Pork, wheat, corn syrup, rice, certain mushrooms, dead salt, and cooked flesh are foods that cause people to have characteristic L-formed acid-fast cell-wall deficient bacteria in the blood for some time after ingesting them.

Altered states of consciousness naturally open up abilities within the body to unleash unused and unrealized talents that enhance immunity and help transform already consumed foodstuff. For conditions relating to joint function, about 50 percent of the cause can be attributed to a stiff state of mind, and 50 percent a need for sufficient levels of Vitamin E to balance the enzyme hyaluronidase, which is involved in swelling synovial sheaths of joints. Very often the person is dehydrated, adding to the condition. Additionally, colloidal minerals and an efficient heavy metal-removal program may be needed.

Microscopic observation of living blood can show signs of a need for various vitamins. Red blood cells can be spiculated (thorny, helmet shaped); blood cells can also be stacked up and enlarged, linked, or rouleaved. With proper nutrition some of these conditions can be cleared in minutes.

Thrombocytes and L-formed bacteria do not allow bioelectromagnetic/gravitic forces to flow correctly. Cells require an integral electrostatic valence for vital functioning. Cells are vitalized and devitalized by a steady stream of electricity, or by its depletion. Colloidal substrates of ellagic acid are found as whole food complexes, such as those found in the herb black walnut, which stimulates nerve force while disassembling unhealthy (dysbiotic) bacteria. Eco-sterilizing life colloids produce substances that are the same ones manufactured by plants for the same purpose. Mytansine, a powerful anti-cancer phytochemical, can be isolated from microorganisms.

Properties of colloidal substrate phytochemicals can be used to calm a person down, and also as an antidote for venomous snakebites! Herbal interferons from the herb lobelia removes warts and pimples and has great power to remove obstructions when supported by other herbs and proper hygiene and lifestyle patterns. Nordihydroguaiaretic acid (NDGA), from the herb chaparral, has various powerful antioxidant properties that act in healthy blood to block electron transport, denying pleomorphic organisms electrical energy required for their survival.

Virus spores are large molecules with interesting geometric shapes that generally have about twenty sides, like herpes. The overall size of a herpes spore is 150 to 200 nm (nanometer = 0.000000001 of a meter). Spores of the identified herpes family are characteristically greasy and totally saturated with lipids from rancid fats.

The key to an alkaline- and oxygen-vital body is LifeFood—and enzymes are the most integral piece. Metabolism of a nutrient is based on water solubility. Fats and lipids and allied vitamins like Vitamins A and E must be broken down. Lipids and fats are emulsified and made miscible by being combined with a colloidal protein envelope. Enzymes make all of this possible. Fat-soluble and already in a water-soluble form, vitamins are absorbed efficiently with LifeFood because they possess a full complement of enzymes. Otherwise, large particles resist absorption.

Enzymes, Immunity, and the Magic Wand

Blood doesn't always maintain its discreet isotonic state. Red blood cells can be clumped and stacked as platelets aggregate together. Blood is the actual working element in the body and enzymes do the work of biologically transmutating and maintaining vital body tissue and fluid pH. Enzymes are very pH sensitive! Large substrates are reduced and cleared by numerous enzymes that transmutate various parts of the substrate simultaneously. Enzymes break down and biologically transmutate adhesion molecules.[35] Intrinsic enzymes can differentiate between adhesion molecules of healthy cells and neoplastic cells, which are cancerous. Health restoration requires a vital enzyme system to maintain body pH.

Good immunity requires enzymes. A compromised immunity is restored with the powerful work of enzymes because immune complexes[36] are transmutated. Immunity works best as immune complexes are cleared from the blood. Therapeutic healing modalities should be directed at the body's immuno-pathological process. This constitutes a biological rather than chemical response.

LifeFood Nutritional Fasting[37] is an effective immune-aiding and building ally, and is the ideal way to heal the body. Proteolytic enzymes activate macrophages and NK (Natural Killer) lymphocyte cells[38] by clearing immune complexes. Enzymes induce beneficial immune mediators for inflammation control that include Tumor Necrosis Factor (TNF), which is produced by immune cells, and other body cells to dissolve haywire cancer cells. Neoplastic cytokines[39] are produced by immune scavenger cells (macrophages). Cachectin is a polypeptide produced and released by macrophages that lyse cells. In an out-of-balance body, cachaxia is a condition of unchecked autolysis that creates wasting-away syndrome. Again, enzymes are vitally needed here to balance the system no matter which way it leans. Hydrolytic/proteolytic enzymes cleave to polymerized TNF and interlock to inactivate and dissolve tumors. Fibrinolytic enzymes limit clot formation.

Oral enzymes (from a good source—a broad-spectrum digestive enzyme tablet, or powder, will split protein, fat, carbohydrates, sugar, and dairy) and coordinated movement of bodily systems allow for perfect shape and right size and number of blood cells. Enzymes in LifeFood and a general sense of well being alter blood platelet shape to increase microcirculation. Enzymes are vitally important anti-inflammatory agents.

CHAPTER 7

Spontaneous Remission

Peple who have difficulty with blood sugar regulation, neoplastic cell lysing, cardio-vascular efficiency, joint ease of motion, nerve protection, integrity of body immunity, and all other health challenges, and who have had a spontaneous remission of their symptoms, experience the lifting of the veil of illusion and provide examples of nature's great healing power. You are nature and as such your body is a perfect self-correcting mechanism when given the proper resources. Listen carefully and open up. Nature wants to heal you if you'll give yourself a chance. If you take the time to evoke a cleansing reaction, time to rest and allow the body's own curative mechanisms to be harnessed, the debris in the body will be cleared away.

We've found that spontaneous remission occurs when at least two of the three (some say four) aspects of ourselves become engaged in change that usually comes with a great amount of deep inner moral inventory. These aspects are: 1) spiritual, 2) emotional, and 3) physical, and possibly 4) mental. Our work with remission primarily involves an active change toward healthy habits with at least two of the spiritual, emotional, or physical aspect of ourselves.

For instance, a person confronted with a cancer diagnosis may take a deep personal inventory and find that they have an utter disgust or extreme dissatisfaction with some aspects of their life. Are they living their sacred contract out and making heaven on Earth, or simply putting in hard time on planet Earth? Perhaps this inner glance reveals a pattern of cutting off powerful emotions rather than feeling them and getting to the other side of them. This block may have led to being non-emotive and rather cold toward other people. They may find that a driving force in their lives, perhaps career goals or motherhood, becomes a convenient excuse for avoiding unpleasant, yet important, emotional, physical, or spiritual work.

It's fairly common for a client to come to David or me looking for a physical solution to an emotional or spiritual issue. They want an herbal recommendation to correct a life-long pattern of not connecting emotionally with their sexual partner. They want a vitamin to correct the fact that they sit in a chair and stare at a computer for ten hours a day. There are many things that will help these symptoms—including herbs and vitamins—that will, if nothing else, raise the person's electrical field to clear their head so they can make wiser choices for themselves. But these things are not solutions to the root causes of the issue. Sure, it's important to add extra nutrients to directly deal with your nutritional demands. If you smoke or work in a polluted environment, for instance, it's important to take extra antioxidants, such as Vitamin C or pyctnogenals to compensate. If you have a stressful life or rely purely on brainpower for your work, you'll want to take extra magnesium to compensate. However, what is the root cause? It is so important to establish the root cause for symptoms to really nail an effective treatment. Whether physical, emotional, spiritual, and mental—all symptoms are a nested matrix of these four aspects of us. How we feel about what we do and who we do it with can lift our mood and boost our immune system, and likewise, it can destroy us. The emotional component is powerful beyond words.

Back to spontaneous remission, let's say that this person decides to evoke a change in diet to LifeFood and creates a powerful healing response. She also confronts her emotional component with bold and courageous passion for the truth of it. These two factors—physical and emotional—can be enough to bring about a spontaneous remission.

This can go dozens of different ways, of course, as many ways as the human spirit can divine, an infinite number. A person may have a powerful spiritual experience that lights up one's memory of Spirit and one's connection to all things. One may couple this with a new habit of exercise and a commitment to eat more LifeFood.

How we feel about our work and what we do for a living is crucial to having a measure of satisfaction in our lives. Longevity of life with a nice body and good mental condition require an attunement to inner principles and desires. When you love what you do, it's like heaven on Earth. When you disrespect the work you do it's putting in hard time on planet Earth. Humans have a peculiar trait that is unique among all other life forms. We are more likely to die on Monday mornings than on any other day of the week at any other time. Rather than die on Friday evening before a nice weekend with the family, the vast majority of people stay around for the enjoyment of their lives—their weekend—and leave this lifetime before going through another awful week doing a job that they don't care about with people they perhaps don't respect. The words, "I'd rather die now than live another week at this job," are a very real phenomenon. Are you working for a living, or living for your work? Do you love what you do and how you spend your day?

People do heal from supposedly incurable conditions; maybe you've heard of someone who went into remission. History books are full of them. There's many examples of the HIV+ person who made love hundreds of times without passing it on to their partner. It couldn't be that HIV is only transmitted through sexual contact because there are hundreds of cases where that is not the case at all. The manifestation of AIDS or HIV, or any other disease, must include malnutrition and drug abuse, recreational and pharmaceutical drugs, and most especially antibiotics abuse, and other toxic chemicals, that break down the immune system. There are so many examples of people living in the midst of disease and virulent viruses that have survived. Secrets of an alkaline body explains why this is so and how to boost your own immune system.

We hope this message restores your feeling of having options in your life. We've worked with many "terminal" clients who had dramatic recoveries. David and I have a broad background in the psychosomatic interplay of mind and body and the use of hypnosis; we understand how belief systems are formed and how this can either aid someone or devastate their condition, depending on how they view their situation. The labels of disease are labels of a static negative; they are not positive and moving. Spontaneous remission is a sweet, innocent event owing to nature's ability to heal from within.

What is this mechanism of miraculous healing? For most people this ability remains untapped. Why is so much research money going into drugs and surgeries when spontaneous healing is a possibility? There is also the greater puzzle as to how it's possible that doctors and the cancer research/pharmaceutical industry money machine can be completely blind to spontaneous remission and its mechanisms, or even the compelling evidence of the placebo effect. Since the early 1970s there have been more people making a living off of cancer than those dying from it. This must play a role in the trend to ignore certain evidence.

Colloidal biology can give you the keys to understand true secrets of health and to become more self-actualized. This is a crash course, which integrates each of the disciplines and allows one who is a good servant to others to heal through the realization of this important avenue of investigation.

Spontaneous Remission Therapeutics (SRT)

David and I have always shown great interest in extensive and intensive investigations of the events that occur when someone has spontaneous remission from a long-standing ailment. Out of the joy of being a good servant, many of the answers to these mechanisms are answered through the process of these investigations. Although we skim over the psychosomatic aspect of spontaneous remission for the purposes of this book, we have written about it at length and those interested should see our website for upcoming publications in the field. Here we will focus on the physical mechanism. Physiologically, remission is a basic condition that is triggered in the body by a state of autolysis. A person's lifestyle and habits have to be altered and the body's curative powers within harnessed and directed through LifeFood Nutritional Fasting and organ and tissue cleansing. This is the key to an extended life. Practitioners of alternative medicine see spontaneous remission more commonly than their standard medicine counterparts for obvious reasons. One of the major reasons is the biological revolution now underway in alternative medicine. We are on the threshold of a petrochemical paradigm that is changing and on its way out. Petrochemicals are in so many modern products; they suppress our immunological response and cause the body's immunological response to be challenged, compromising the immune system's restorative powers.

We long to see the day when the green grocer will be required to post the long list of chemicals—the pesticide, herbicide, fungicide, and xeno-estrogens—that commercially grown produce contains. If you knew what it commercial produce were sprayed with, would you eat it? Who would buy it? You will reach for the produce that is grown organically, or better yet, biodynamically. Did you know that organically grown greens possess up to 85 percent more nutrients than the bland, pale, poisoned, and gassed commercially grown produce? Organically grown food generally has two to three times the vitamin, minerals, and trace elements of commercially grown food. If it's not in the soil, air, or water then it won't be in the food. Organic food has higher quality nutritional properties that offer the body a vast array of excellent quality building materials. After all, you are what you eat.

Most diseases must attain a certain critical mass for the body condition to be on the threshold of immune inhibition. Immunity becomes activated and boots out any foreign proteins at the sign of threat to the body's health; the system becomes fresh again the moment debris is flushed and cleared out of the system. It is as simple as that! Colloidal biology defines this part of our immune system, which refuses to be inhibited. This is about both a primitive and new immune system.

What is it about one person's immune response that is completely resistant to carcinogens, whereas another person falls prey to the chief undertakers—mold, fungus, and yeast? The understanding of the principle that proper pH supports life and the realization that the terrain is everything, dates back through the history of medical ancestry, through a line of dedicated people who understood pleomorphism. This is a pure and natural therapeutic involving biology that has dramatic results where none in petrochemical allopathy previously existed.

It's inspiring to see people who suffer with pneumonia, chronic fatigue syndrome, or high Polymerase Chain Reaction (PCR) counts improve dramatically upon following a few days of cleansing. They get to witness the miracle transpire as they actually witness themselves feeling gradually better. We have seen people with full-blown AIDS heal enlarged lymph nodes and low T4 and high T8 cell counts and go into remission. We have helped educate many people as to how to care for themselves and watched them achieve dramatic results. This goes for raising animal immunity as well as healing all manner of degenerative diseases.

Spontaneous remission occurs as the body clears debris away and makes hormones and minerals available to cells through an enzymatic process. This is what the body needs in order to mount and control an inflammation and to help respire colloidal body tissue integrity. There are life colloids that can live only within a certain environment; so the moment that the body serum is clean these life colloids wash and penetrate deep into the liver. Within three weeks every single cell of the liver is built of high-integrity material.

Doctors may mistake the response as having come from a specific organism rather than as a result of the body's own ability to clear away debris and move forward with the natural inflammatory response. Antibiotics, and all kinds of pharmaceuticals, inhibit a true immune response. As you apply biology in healing there are a surprising number of techniques and modalities that help eliminate foreign tissue, both benign and malignant, and cast out debris. The life colloids (somatids, spores, and double spores) are an important modality to disassemble cancer cells (mold and fungal forms). We use LifeFood nutrition to employ immunoglobulins to tag tumorous foreign protein deposits in the body and clear these obstructions out. The immunoglobulins anti-genically mark cancerous cells that draw the forces of local immunity in the manner of inflammation that disassemble, or lyse, tagged foreign cellular debris.

There are life colloids found in certain fungi that have a high affinity for neoplastic cancer cells that, with their fungal filaments, completely disassemble colloids that are perfectly inert to healthy cells. In the presence of LifeFood and a healthy body terrain, less than healthy cells yield, change, and become normal. These cells also respond positively when the brain is in proper resonance and the body is given its food in the form of whole food vitamin mineral colloids. Various plant-derived chemicals help target incurable conditions of the body, such as bacterial infections, when combined with tissue cleansing. As always, it is imperative to maintain good hygiene practices, both internally and externally. Eat clean food and keep your body clean—especially hands and fingernails. The most virulent bacteria found on the body is under the fingernails, where people pick up toxins by touching their teeth, lips, eyes, ears, and nose. This is called autointoxification. Simply keeping the hands and nails scrubbed allows mycotoxins to completely pass you by. Wash your hands regularly with a gentle all-natural soap with few ingredients.

We apply an understanding of chelation therapies that target, tag, and clean. This is the process of nature's powerful healing. Body cells that have broken down into smaller conglomerates of colloids, such as pieces of DNA or RNA, resonate, and through their resonance cause cells that are out of harmony to also lyse apart into the sizes of viral spore forms that can become bacterial forms like staphylococcus. We have witnessed people respond beautifully when educated as to how to care for themselves through LifeFood Nutrition.

We have seen people heal who were given a prognosis of only a few weeks to live. They are living today, healed of neoplastic cells. Their health vitality has changed forever. This process for most people requires at least a year and a half of tissue cleansing for the more stubborn conditions; however, most everyone receives benefits from only a few days. This information should be used to educate yourself and take personal responsibility in your life; develop a proper lifestyle that supports your immune system and the environment.

We allow the body to prepare itself to cleanse and heal stagnant organs and body tissue. We stimulate the body to go into a state of autolysis whereby the blood chemistry begins to dissolve and penetrate tumors, cysts, and all tissue that needs to be rejuvenated, thus overcoming the body's threshold inhibition. Tissue cleansing and LifeFood Nutrition radically alter the terrain, allowing it to become clear and clean. We use LifeFood Nutritional Fasting to debulk the body.

Debulking the gut causes the body to overcome tumor threshold inhibition in a way that allows the immune system to wake up and use inner healing forces. People have to wake up and put something fresh into their body each day. Restoring the option of life is coming about as a result of people's connectedness to the Earth. This is a big shift from the guy in a white lab coat with a sad stern face talking to you about your medical condition. Yikes! A diagnosis from this guy could be scary—enough to cause some trauma on its own.

Giving you the option of life by using food as medicine will restore vitality, getting you back on this side of the bell curve. A fresh LifeFood smoothie consumed for lunch or between meals has glycos-amino-glycans (GAGs) and an assortment of lignans derived from plants. With its broad spectrum of absorbable nutrition, a LifeFood smoothie can serve as a truly wonderful option to help people debulk and reduce left-behind meals from years past, while flooding in electrons that blast through nerve pathways. Plus, they taste really great. Once you've had LifeFood, you'll never be able to feel the same way toward dead food again. Your taste buds become educated to what real food tastes like and you'll be able to eliminate dead food flavors like rancid oil in your cupboard. Your taste becomes much more refined in this way.

People who get onto LifeFood and begin to tissue cleanse for one or two months realize a dramatic improvement toward better health. Overall, you will see an increase in energy, improved blood vitality, and qualitative change in body composition (muscle to fat). Phytochemical nutrients in LifeFood promote a healthy terrain, which dissolves neo-plastic cells in many ways. It's unfortunate that so many diets are put together by people who don't understand the metaphysical nature of the body. Let's take a closer look at some of the ingredients in LifeFood Nutrition.

LifeFood Ingredients to Better Health

With LifeFood, every single ingredient is presented to the body in its whole food vitamin/mineral complex form. We recommend that people use whole flax seed, either freshly ground or soaked. There is a great deal of research about oil and protein combinations. Later we go into the importance of essential fatty acids (EFAs) that are bound to sulfur-rich proteins. However, LifeFood and cold-pressed oil are made miscible in the body fluid, allowing important essential fatty acids to be properly assimilated. Fresh living oil, like coconut butter and flaxseed oil, are good for you because they make the blood slippery and greatly enhance brain performance. We recommend three tablespoons of good cold-pressed living oil each day for everyone.

Through the 14-Day LifeFood Nutritional Fast, a person clears away starch/mucous adhesions and stones from the liver, gall bladder, intestine, and from the entire digestive system. The fast also provides the body essential fatty acids through consuming good oil/protein combinations. We have witnessed people who had yellowish-green bile pigment replaced with healthy red pigment in the blood. Lipoprotein reappears spontaneously and phosphotids return in remission.

One of the more vital elements of nutrition are essential fatty acids. In nearly all blood studies just about everyone shows an utter and devastating lack of EFAs. Albumin and phosphotids in LifeFood Nutrition combine flax seed oil and sulfur-rich proteins, found in our raw blended LifeFood soups, which enable EFAs to become completely soluble. LifeFood is electron-rich and causes membranes of our lattice to become more stable, which makes our body more flexible and fluid. The blood becomes more slippery and the entire vascular system becomes very elastic. This gives the skin snap. It cleans up the bloodstream flow by loosening and particalizing silt left from starches and carts it out. LifeFood's electron-rich EFAs allow the body the most amazing transportation of materials and allow an energy exchange between the inside and outside of the cell membrane. It's imperative we impart how important this process is in restoring vitality to cells and having good immunity.

Let's delve into essential fatty acids a little more because they are so important. They are very active biological substances that help us produce prostaglandins. EFAs are similar substances to the hormones that are produced locally by cells. Omega-3 essential fatty acids supply the precursors to make prostaglandins. These substances are involved in nearly every bodily function! Tumor suppression is promoted by protiglandins E2 by increasing protiglandins E3. Gama Linolenic Acid (GLA) and other oils have been found to dissolve (necrose) cancerous neoplasms in the body, and also in lab research using tumor cell lines. Studies show a significant reduction in neoplastic growth in animals that were fed proper levels of omega-3 essential fatty acids.

Freshly ground flax seed contains rich lignans and precursors of elements needed for a broad spectrum of biological activity, including lysing neoplastic cells and clearing foreign spores from the body. This simple seed, the flax seed, has benefited many women in relieving symptoms of menopause and restoring temperature regulation. The active ingredient in flax seed that relieves these symptoms is the phytochemical coumariac acid.

Flax seed lignans are converted into various steroid-like compounds that take part in helping the body maintain vital tissue integrity and clearing foreign proteins. LifeFood Nutrition has an array of plant steroid-like compounds that block estrogens—a neoplastic promoting effect. Lipotropic factors, amino acids, essential fatty acids, and a variety of colloidal minerals are all available in the flax seed. Flax seed is an integral food used for medicine in the LifeFood program's tissue cleansing.

To give away a few more secrets about the super smoothie (see recipe in Appendix): the blue-green algae/spirulina/chlorella in it has an enormous amount of protein (80 percent)! It's loaded with Vitamins B, C, and E and contains mucopolysaccharides plus omega-3 EFAs. There are colloidal elements in blue-green algae/spirulina/chlorella that improve immune ability. This has been demonstrated even in people who have been exposed to Agent Orange, mustard gas, chemotherapy, and radiation treatment. By the way, chemotherapy is very similar to Agent Orange molecularly.

There are elements in blue-green algae macrophage activity that help the ill body go into remission and shrink tumors. Interferon production is stimulated in the body, providing phytochemicals that help repair DNA. Blue-green algae also contains significant GAGs (carbohydrates linked to a core protein). There are steroid-like compounds found abundantly in LifeFood that help moderate cholesterol and lower viscous blood fats, while strengthening the tissue of our body and keeping it anchored together in a good way. Certain LifeFood has phytochemicals with estrogenic properties that can block estrogen's effect and stimulate neoplastic cells to lyse. These phytochemicals cause cells to de-differentiate. Those cells become more primitive and eventually lyse.

Isoflavanoids help regulate the body's hormonal system and help relieve symptoms of menopause and prostate conditions. David and I would like to keep things simple here, rather than give you a taxonomy of phytochemicals and their properties in health. Suffice it to say that a broad and varied diet rich in LifeFood delivers a stream of plant-based nutrients to the body that are easy to assimilate—for fuel, hygiene, and high-integrity materials.

LifeFood Stops Cancer in Its Tracks and Clears Clogged Arteries

We have had great success with people who experience remission of cancer. Lemons and grapefruit are used extensively in remission, prepared in electrolyte beverages. Our signature beverage, *Electrolyte Lemonade,* is a fresh, raw lemonade with a little oil and salt (see recipe in Appendix). *Electrolyte Lemonade* modifies the citrus pectin for absorption into lymph. Elements of this citrus pectin are absorbed through the lymph to become bound to the surface of PC (immune) cells that go to work to protect cells from metastatic neoplastic cancerous conditions. Pectin-bound free-floating neoplastic cells are slippery and unable to anchor to any tissue, thus more easily eliminated from the body. Unhealthy neoplastic growth is found when colloids have the ability to pierce the membranes that protect the body tissue. The chief undertakers—mold, fungus and yeast—invade the blood stream and lymphatic system.

Before neoplastic cells can travel from the capillaries into the organs, where secondary forms can then assemble, LifeFood effectively starves the neoplastic cells from having any energy, reversing the state of cancer where neoplastic cells rob the host's organs and vital systems of nutrients. Thus, in the case of remission, we find that the body overcomes neoplastic proliferation. Colloidal integrity of the blood causes our organs to become filtrated with vital rich nutrients that dissolve foreign proteins and allow the body organs to perform essential functions.

Citrus pectin bound with oil is absorbed in the lymph, bypassing the villi of the intestinal route that citric acid would ordinarily take through the intestines. This modified citrus pectin and its high-density lipoprotein lymphatic transportation helps provide enzymes needed for cellular interactions involving cell surface components such as galactoside-binding neoplastic cell membrane anchors called lectins.

Neoplastic cells use adhesion molecules that allow them to connect to red blood (endothelial) cells. Galactins in *Electrolyte Lemonade* bind to lectins. Cancer cells have galacto-seeking proteins on their surface membranes. Lectins are a velcro-like substance that cancer cells use to adhere to endothelial cells, like a blood vessel or an organ, allowing neoplastic cells to colonize. Galactins present in *Electrolyte Lemonade* clear arteriosclerotic plaque and bind to lectins of cancer cells that then are lysed from the body.

GAGs (carbohydrates linked to a core protein) compose highly structured gels that occupy a very large amount of tissue composition in our body, mainly in the connective tissue. These are nutrients with an extremely high negative-density charge.

Hyaluronic acid and other GAGs are responsible for helping lyse some 50 percent of colon and 10 percent of lung and breast neoplastic cells. Hyaluronic acid works by inhibiting cancer cell motility. Hyaluronic acid is part of these neoplastic cell motility. Neoplastic cell membranes have receptors that sit on top of their surface and serve as their ears and eyes. Certain phytochemicals are absolutely crucial for healing; however, we want you to know you already make all of the things you need within your body as long as you keep in good health. Given the body's ability to debulk itself and improve internal and external hygiene, you can get back on the growing side of the bell curve through the steps we lay out in LifeFood Nutrition.

A person may have a degree of robustness even if they are carrying around a wad of fat around their jowls, gut, and thighs—the evidence of left over meals and years of glutinous behavior. Are you living to eat, or eating to live? Be more alive in your life with LifeFood Nutrition and consider the benefit of cellular cleansing. It generally takes a year and a half to restore a person back to good order.

People needing to clear pleomorphic organisms and neoplastic cells from the body are encouraged to use a course of action that robs electrons from those life forms. LifeFood Nutrition and tissue cleansing selectively block all unfriendly life colloids and lyse them away while at the same time easily feeding healthy cells. Let's take a look at a few LifeFood nutrients.

Lecithin, an ingredient in the nutmilk and super smoothie in our program, is integral in assisting the liver to detoxify, rebuild, and correct phospholipid functioning and its production. Neoplastic cells and pleomorphic cells consume sugar at a far greater rate than other cells, robbing from the liver. A person can block this energy source and induce the body to derive energy generated from fats rather than sugars. Hydroxy citric acid, DHEA, and other nutrients also help block glucose 6 phosphate dehydrogeninase 6 dehydrogenaise (G6PD enzyme) that convert sugar to fat causing the body cells to burn fat in the Krebs cycle.

Remission occurs as pleomorphic and neoplastic life colloids are starved from blood sugar. Refined sugar feeds tumors. Elevated blood sugar diverts prostaglandin pathways toward tumor promotion (PGE—2). This prostaglandin is immuno-suppressive and clumps blood cells; it causes vascular-constriction and practically inhibits the biosynthetic pathways of estrogen binders.

Remission requires selectively maintaining low levels of blood sugar. We educate people about LifeFood and the remarkable difference between living food and hybridized food. Hybrid foods demand insulin production. Insulin over-production from eating hybrid food taxes the pancreas and liver, a problem that has become so chronic in our society it has borne a whole new range of diseases called insulin-resistance disease. A person on LifeFood will produce very little insulin because there isn't any need for it.

Medium chain oils (MCTs) from flax seed oil and coconut butter keep blood sugar levels low. These foods are a very easy source of energy for healthy cells. Neoplastic cells, on the other hand, require up to fifteen times more sugar. Central nervous system tumors are generally fed by glucose that causes cachaxia (wasting away).

Neoplastic cells draw sugar from the liver by converting lactic acid into glucose. The protocol we recommend is to inhibit neoplastic gluco-neo-genesis while allowing normal cell metabolism to grow. An important component of the LifeFood program is holding back the body mechanisms of cachaxia along with helping the body dissolve neoplastic cells—*like snowballs on a hot plate!*

Various cell nutrients from marine minerals, mistletoe, celandine, goat whey, seed cheese, colostrum, tocotreinols, and lecithin help provide biologically active globular proteins to the body that coat pathogens for clearing by the immune system (opsonize). Micronutrients help the body do enumerable other things aside from the very important task of enhancing gastrointestinal colonization. LifeFood is packed with enzymes that have anti-spore, anti-pleomorphic, and anti-parasitic function and that keep the body hygienic and naturally eco-sterilized. To keep the digestive tract in good order we recommend L. Salivarius, or L. Planitarium, or another good probiotic or kyo-dophilus bacteria blend to promote healthy bacteria.

A couple of other nutrients that help protect epithelial cells of the lungs, stomach, skin, and pancreas are carotenoids (red, green, and yellow pigments) and phycocyaninines (blue pigments). Carotenoids enhance T and B lymphocyte proliferative responses along with T and NK lymphocyte tumorcidal capacity. Fresh raw almond butter is alkaline-forming and has benzaldehyde (Vitamin B17). We recommend enzymes, too, of course. Enzymes help with fat digestion so the liver has plenty of essential fatty acids. We especially encourage sulfur-bearing amino acids and sulfur-rich foods, like cabbages with their amazing healing power. Cabbages contain Vitamin U that is essential for healthy intestinal function. The amino acid glutamine helps thicken digestive cells, is a fuel for immune cells and the brain, and helps conserve the liver's antioxidants.

Proteolytic enzymes are integral to good health. We combine the antioxidant herb turmeric with the enzyme bromelain. Bromelain helps spare elements in the turmeric cause the body to have phytochemical power, which activate key nutrients in the plasma responsible for the breakdown of fibrin. Deconstructing fibrin is key for disarming receptors on the surface of neoplastic cells. Neoplastic cells and pleomorphic life colloids in the body develop excessive fibrin, causing poor blood flow and fibrous blockages in the connective fiber of the body. Neoplastic cells use fibrin as a camouflage.

A glyco-protein shield compromises the body's ability to completely lyse neoplastic cells. Stimulating the process of autolysis promotes the debulking of the body to stimulate remission of symptoms. Turmeric has proteolytic enzymes that act as anti-coagulant and fibrolytic agent that helps lyse the colloids of the neoplastic fibrin coating, allowing the vital immune system to lyse those neoplastic cells. Bromelain inhibits neoplastic growth by blocking production of mucus that ordinarily protects the surface of neoplastic cells. This allows lymphatic cells to dock to neoplastic cells, helping them to be cleared up. It also inactivates PGE-2s. In the fresh, raw soup recipes in the *LifeFood Recipe Book*, the onions, broccoli, and blue-green algae have flavon quercetin, a substance known to powerfully block tumors and pro-flammatory reactions.

Your Liver Is Your Genie in a Bottle

Detoxification of the blood and body is owed primarily to the liver. The liver is the body's sewage treatment plant. The liver neutralizes and removes poisons from the blood and synthesizes various compounds. This vital responsibility is accomplished through enzymes specially equipped by the liver. You could say liver tissue is an intestinal venous drainage filter and factory.

Bile neutralizes acid churn from the stomach to activate fat/lipid and carbohydrate enzymes and emulsify lipid/fat in the small intestine. Bile happens to be the excrement of the liver! About three quarts (1.5 liters) of bile pour forth daily from the liver, peaking at 3 P.M. regardless of what's been eaten. The role of liver detoxification is vital to keeping the blood and body clean. Blood profiles often have measures of biological indicators revealing liver function.

The liver organizes great regeneration powers; hygiene enhances liver rejuvenation powers. Spores are the spent material of lysed proteins from various tissue that became inflamed due to toxins and low levels of anionic[40] elements.

Lavish eating can require an outpouring of alkaline elements to neutralize acids and activate digestive and assimilative enzymes. Insipid puss from overly acid body tissue is positively charged and cholesterol salts bind to this puss to form gall bladder and intestinal adhesions, resulting in the inefficient functioning of the liver.

Stone formation and dissolvability depend upon the composition of the bile. High cholesterol demand for bile flow, under the influence of over-acidity, causes cholesterol stones to form. When bile acids decrease and cholesterol increases crystals form and grow to become gravel, which fuses to make larger stones. Stones also form because of the liver's inability to handle abnormal necrosis of blood cells (hemolysis).

The liver is typically the first organ to restore and is arguably the most important organ for many reasons. With over one hundred functions, the liver produces factors that regulate clotting.

The liver regulates many body functions through the manufacturing of various enzymes. Liver cells are relatively indistinguishable from one another because they are quite fine. Superconduction across its liquid crystal cell membranes reveals temperature sensitivity. In a healthy liver we find a perpetual flow of electrons with a magnetic field brought about by electrons spinning as they wobble in their orbit. They appear like a cloud around their nucleus through the individualized magnetic fields within each cell.

Life Taps into Free Energy

Subatomic energies of zero-point residuum, pair production, vacuum polarization, and all the forces of the universe are manifest in the liver. With the efficiency of a factory, the liver biologically transmutates one element into another. People have an idea of what malnutrition apparently is from the outside—stick-thin limbs and bloated bellies, listless eyes on blank faces—though less noticeable is malnutrition from the inside, much of which is attributable to what a person eats that causes electrons to be lost.

Prenatal and neonatal malnutrition has resulted in the underdevelopment of the brain and central nervous system of 70 percent of today's population. Where there is adequate nutrition we find good immunity and brain functioning. Electricity is conducted by the flow of ionized mineral colloids. Much of the foodstuff available today is totally devoid of absorbable minerals that can become incorporated into the nucleus of our cells.

It is less commonly realized that those trace elements activate enzymes. Enzymes are required for vitamins to function. Vitamins help absorb minerals. Minerals are more integral to nutrition than basic nutrients, protein, vitamins, fats, and even water; they play a key role even though these other nutrients are unquestionably essential.

Colloidal mineral composition of the cell interior is vigilantly maintained. Even small departures from what is normal simply aren't tolerated. Homeostasis occurs within a threshold between narrow limits of pH, electrical conductivity, and negative redox in the plasma so that the integrity of tissue is safeguarded. For minerals to become miscible with water, it's important that they be drawn into the body fluid where they become linked to protein carriers, mostly albumin.

Colloidal minerals become bound to chelates of amino acids. The mineral usually allows two or maybe three aminos to chelate (dipeptide or tripeptides). Body metabolism is regulated by enzymes that are formed when mineral colloids are naturally chelated by cells. Imbued with bioenergetic fields, it is primarily vitamins, minerals, and amino acids that compose the substance of enzymes. Oxidative enzymes are heat-sensitive.

The liquid crystal membranes of our body have a perpetual flow of electrons, and life possesses the property of energy generation! The body has elements that enable life to produce a net energy output exceeding the total energy input by the enormous incalculable potential energy that is tapped from the environment. What is it about the aloe vera plant that allows it to go on living for quite some time without access to any sunlight? (Or even any soil!) How does life like this aloe vera regenerate itself without light or soil?

Solar, chemical, fluidic, mechanical, nuclear, and thermal energies are tapped by living cells. Cells have their own individualized gravitational magnetic fields and make good use of tachyon energy. Everything is a condensed gradation of cosmic energy. In a healthy body there is a place on the abdomen that is very resonant when percussed. There is the perfect resonation when high colloidal mineral composition integrity gives rise to an energy source that enables superconduction in primitive life colloids and complex life forms.

Biology enjoys superconduction that is typically heat sensitive to the overall amount of electrons collectively needed to survive as a miniature world. Heat causes a release of electrons and cold causes a freezing. We find colloids everywhere; they live within the sun and under extreme temperature in volcanic hot water vents at the bottom of the ocean, as well as within the cooling systems in nuclear reactors. The cells in our body can survive higher temperatures than dysbiotic life forms, thus thermogenics is a form of immunity where dysbiotic life is lysed.

Life forms need a constant supply of electrons. Below or above a critical temperature and resonance threshold there is a state of superconduction. The voltage within the life form is gauged through its ability to be in resonance; it is an energy source that is in resonance within the life form. Perpetual motion of electrons occurs as a management of monatomic colloids provides the life force with a continuous current. This is what colloidal biology is all about.

Magnetic fields created in such a manner can be maintained indefinitely beyond what is ordinary. One can live without eating any solid food for years, just taking in LifeFood beverages. Many of our cancer clients have chosen to do back-to-back 14-Day LifeFood Nutritional Fasts for six months to a year, until their tumors were gone and they felt completely rejuvenated. Huge tumors shrink in this way. It doesn't really matter where they are in the body, or what the condition is—heart disease, fibroids, fibromyalgia, lymphoma, or any other physical symptoms gathered under a name to be called a disease.

A disease is really just a group of symptoms, and it's a shame that so much attention is given to the disease rather than healing its symptoms one by one. In allopathic medicine a treatment is prescribed when the disease is identified; this "cookbook" approach to medicine replaces true medical healing for a band-aid cure that is mostly limited to pharmaceutical drugs and surgery. Though they can be lifesavers in trauma injuries, drugs and surgery used to treat disease as a band-aid approach to healing is truly dangerous. Rather than track the symptoms down to their roots and healing the body from there, hospitals today require that the person's illness be identified and named in order to appease the insurance companies that demand it. Even if your symptoms don't neatly fit under a particular disease title, hospitals and doctors will diagnose you in order to get insurance companies to approve a therapy or treatment that they deem worthy enough to pay for. The insurance companies have an enormous amount of power in the medical profession and often have the last word on what treatment you can have, regardless of what you would like or what may be best for you.

David and I used to like chatting with my uncle before he passed over a few years ago. He was one of only two Washington State auditors for hospitals. He worked his way around the state auditing one hospital after another, and he found the same thing in the billing practices of every hospital without exception. They all had a conscious pattern of over-billing and double-billing the client and the client's insurance program. The hospital would send the client a bill that wasn't itemized but rather just a lump sum. The client submits it to their insurance company, which tells them how much is their share. Then the hospital sends out another bill for some itemized costs, say a $500 bill for diagnostic work. The person assumes that this bill is not covered by their insurance plan and writes a check directly to the hospital. The hospital keeps an enormous slush fund account with this double-billed money. The process is a lot more elaborate than I describe here; however, this practice is common all over the country. You have rights and can demand an itemized list of your expenses from any hospital visit. This system needs to be cleaned up, making room for a true healing therapeutic system to emerge. America is one of the richest countries in the world and yet we have the highest obesity rate, cancer and heart disease in the world. We consume more drugs and have more surgery than any other country, and we call ourselves a free country? Freedom is not some lofty doctrine; freedom is having a healthy body and a beautiful environment that is clean and rich in the bounty of nature.

Gallbladder removal surgery is one of the most scheduled surgeries in hospitals today. We have never spoken to someone who has had their gallbladder removed that was given any nutritional recommendations at all. Not even one. No clue as to where or when or how these gallstones showed up, it must be the fault of the gallbladder; let's yank that offensive defective organ out. Yes, that will solve everything; now go on with your life. This surgery is often completely unnecessary. It is a disgraceful lack of understanding of the human body and its healing mechanisms. Our gallbladder flush is a more effective solution for gallbladder ailments, and even for many other chronic conditions and especially as preventative medicine. I was in London last year when I picked up a local newspaper. One story caught my eye: a young woman, only twenty-four years old, had died in the hospital a few days after having elective surgery to remove her otherwise healthy gallbladder that had stones. Her doctor had recommended she have the surgery now rather than later as she was planning to be married in the fall. Like so many hospital experiences, she died from an infection, probably staph, rather than her original condition that wasn't chronic at all. A young girl cut down in her youth with her marriage and life ahead of her. Four or five gallbladder flushes probably would have done the trick. Larry Dossey, M.D., an expert in psychosomatic medicine and a nationally and internationally renowned physician, says that 225,000[41] people die each year from hospital care rather than the disease symptoms they were admitted for. According to Dossey, "This makes hospital care the third leading cause of death in the United States, behind heart disease and cancer."

Most people check into the hospital with an enormous amount of fecal debris in their colon. It would stand to reason that everyone should get a good enema or colonic when they check in to begin the first stage of cleansing—activating the organs of elimination. By the way, before the pharmaceutical paradigm we are presently fighting our way out of, an enema was standard practice upon hospital admittance, and it still is in many countries. Even someone who is there for trauma like a car wreck will benefit from this. Trauma can cause a person to be constipated for days, often because they are injured and cannot make it to the bathroom. I've spoken to many patients who broke bones and were in the hospital for a week and didn't have a bowel movement the entire time! No one even asked! David and I fast regularly. We have also put many thousands of people on fasting programs. We've given the message and tools of fasting and proper care for the body to people who have tried it for themselves and so convinced themselves that it works that they became hooked on it through their own experience. When we flood the body with colloidal minerals by drinking nutmilk or eating a raw LifeFood soup the body goes to work to make good use of them. Again, the body is a perfect self-correcting mechanism. Only a few days on a LifeFood fast gives the person heart to continue on. Every week we receive calls from people who are up and on their feet again because they gave nature a chance.

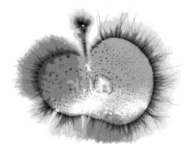

CHAPTER 8

Current Affairs

Immortal Timeless Cycles

Enormous sea turtles can live 600 years. Trees can live thousands of years and somatids (life colloids) can live billions of years, perhaps indefinitely. Atoms possess internal perpetual motion that is enormous. The perpetual rotating motion of electrons around their atomic nuclei gives us the ability to defy gravity and the law of thermodynamics. We are lighter while we have life! The instant we die, the body becomes heavier. The degree of life that we feel today can be measured in our steps and how many pounds of pressure we create when we walk.

You may remember the 1970s TV show "Kung Fu." In the opening credits the protagonist is shown going through the various initiation rites to become a master. In one, he must walk over rice paper and leave no footprints. This is a good example of physical mastery. A Kung Fu master, in this case, has refined his understanding of weight, gravity, and his own electromagnetic field to harness his light body. A true awareness of the light body is usually refined through great discipline and willpower, and following one of the many doctrines where this training is outlined such as martial arts, yoga, shamanism, Tao, and others. This lightening of the body changes during a normal day, usually with our emotions.

We don't have to become martial arts masters to pay attention to how heavily or lightly we pass over the ground. David and I led hundreds of firewalks at our residential trainings during the 1980s and 1990s. This is a fairly simple way to give people an example of how light they can make their body, plus it is very empowering. Walking over red-hot coals and being unscathed tends to pop old paradigms of limitation. Plus, it's nice to be so close to fire without experiencing fear or harm. Of course, there is a bit of a science to running a safe firewalk, and we were meticulous to guarantee the safety of our clients.

Alkalinity equals more electrons. Acidic strength is measured by how empty we are on our electron reserve. We can harness the perpetual motion of electrons in life. Enzymes are imbued with this energy, 95 percent of which creates the magnetic field of every life form and is supplied by the spinning motion of electrons (ferro magnetism). Electron orbit is diamagnetism.[42] Life colloids assemble into angstrom-sized colloidal filaments that act as wave guides for electrons.

Life colloids live within more complex life forms that are in perpetual motion. Absolute zero exists at zero-point energetics, though it is without a specific locale, only a vague notion of existing inside as a life force. This is carried within each life form. All random energy fluctuations are tapped into and given out freely as energy.

Experiments show that an ordinary body cell can live indefinitely beyond its regular one year lifespan if cell fluid is replaced daily. The cell lines used in labs for cancer research for decades are from a single person, a woman who lived during the 1950s. Her cells are still being grown throughout the world. In another experiment, chicken cells have been kept living for twenty-eight years.[43] These cells appear to be almost immortal as long as their waste is removed and they receive proper nutrients.

Artificial Flavorings and Antisocial Behavior

You could say that the last fifty years has been an enormous nutritional experiment! We are consuming materials that never before been consumed in the known history of man. People toil in laboratories in white lab coats designing new flavors for everything from children's cereal and candy, to lipstick, to dead denatured frozen dinners that someone will eat. Market studies show that if the flavors are fantastic enough, people will eat cardboard-like foodstuffs that have no nutritional value at all. Many of these artificial flavors are actually designer drugs that trick the sensitive chemical receptors on the tongue into wanting more and more of that drug/artificial flavoring. Years of research go into the development side of these chemicals, but not on the side of their long-term effect on the body. These artificial flavorings seem to wreak havoc on the finer regions of the brain, most particularly the hippocampus and hypothalamus that have to do with regulating social functions, such as hunger/eating cycles, social/antisocial behavior, sexual function, and other complex physical aspects of behavior governed by emotion and instinct.

What price do we pay for this chemical assault to food? What price have we already paid? The freest country in the world has the most people in prison than any other country, per capita, in the world. In Mexico, a life-sentence in prison is considered cruel and inhumane punishment; they feel it goes against the fundamental rights of existence. It reflects some faith in the human spirit to rehabilitate one's behavior and to become a good citizen again

The practice of exterminating poor disempowered people is nothing less than a disgrace. So are one hundred-year jail sentences that offer absolutely no rehabilitation at all. Jail makes hardened criminals out of nonviolent offenders every day in America. America's prisons are extremely dangerous, violent places where brutal rapes and beatings are tolerated. Nutrition plays a key role in America's problems because artificial flavorings are designer drugs, and should be labeled so because of their effect on brain tissue and behavior. It's so silly to witness the media fuss and blitz that surround pharmaceutical companies when they release their fancy public relations programs geared toward herbal supplements that are often artificial flavorings, seasonings, red and green dyes, and more harmful toxins that are known to cause real damage. Yet, these are still on the market and no one complains. So much of what goes on today is as a result of ruthless marketing that ignores facts about food, medicine, and the environment. It's all about swaying public belief, or simply bombarding the public with a lie so consistently that they finally believe it.

A few years ago, David and I gave a talk to a public school in Louisiana. It was a poor district with mostly black students. We were aghast to find that they had three Ritalin feedings a day. Children deemed problematic were recommended for this drugging by their own teachers. The teachers! Since when are teachers qualified to medicate students? The students were put on one, two, or three doses of Ritalin per day. Per day! We went around to each class and casually interviewed the teachers and we found that some teachers had very few kids on the drug feedings, while other teachers had many students on the drug. Now, these are the poorest kids in a very poor school district. Who is paying for this drugging? But these kids don't need Ritalin. Just the opposite, they need to get off the drugs they don't even know they are on—just like they need to get off the artificial flavorings and colorings, food preservatives, and the like. Everyone recovers on the LifeFood diet. The head clears and in a short while the person starts to feel more solid and able to resolve the issues they confront in everyday life.

Having Hollow Bones

As life forms operate within a variable flux of energy, it becomes necessary to tap into intrinsic life force. Fitness is the margin of energy reserve we have above and beyond what is required to operate. Time-forward and time-reverse electrons meet and light is born from matter. Colloidal biology and the secrets of an alkaline body can sustain the life form—sustain it from its own intrinsic power drawn from the polarization of ferromagnetics. Energy is drawn freely from the electrons within us when we pass on. These life colloids continue to exist long after we go. Hair and nails continue to grow for more than a month after we die.

Free-energy is tapped inside a vacuum. Native Americans have a term for this: *having hollow bones*. This teaching is about how to empty the self, rather than being so full of everything. Language patterns can allow emptiness inside, or they can create a multiplicity of things. Tremendous fluctuations of character can be tapped into by the person who lives life by letting go of unimportant matters.

When there is a union inside of you of two perfectly equal and opposite parts, where the heart and mind are connected, you become an instrument for learning. In this state you have as much time in front of you as behind and it seems as if things arrive sooner than they otherwise would. Ions have unique radiation characteristics, especially when compared to conduction electrons. There is an ion-acoustic within the plasma of the body that produces a resonant sound when the body is in vital health and a certain place is percussed. Monatomic elements propagate coherent vacuum polarization and zero-point energetics in healthy vital blood.

Life taps into environmental radiating energy as a result of the resonance it emits and at the same time absorbs. One can feel this in overtone chanting, or as hemisphere synchronization is happening; you have access to a Eureka phenomena. Other techniques are heart and breath synchronization, other meditations, and analogue sculpting.[44]

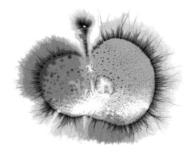

CHAPTER 9

Vitality

Vitality and Superconduction

Tachyons flow within macroscopic lay lines in a continuous manner in the body, without dissipation, with the head (+) and the feet (-) energetically linked by a neutral zone where both flow into each other. The pelvis can accumulate energy when there is tension in the feet and head, and within the neutral zone (pelvis) there can be material that limits circulation. This is a good example of what can happen to cause body temperature to run hot/cold at the poles, beyond temperatures that allow good superconduction within liquid crystal membranes of body cells. State of health in the head, neutral zones, and feet influence the whole body.

Our thoughts can be as important as the energy we get from our food, and as primitive. What thoughts do you have today that will add another day to your life? How relaxed is your face while you eat, work, play, and during other moments? All things in life can be seen as having a positive/negative flow of electrons. Even the language we use can be framed positively, allowing us more access to whole-brain functioning, or can be framed negatively, bringing us into the reptilian parts of the brain.

Life maintains a perpetual magnetic field. Tachyons condense by lines of force in the body when energy is flowing from one pole to the other. For instance, how does your torso resonance at the thyroid negative pole connect with the positive pole of the head? How relaxed is the connective tissue of the stomach? Yoga stretching is good for joint mobility; teaching you to really relax while gaining strength at the same time.

The battery that starts the current, silica, is switched out of the loop after it has assisted in building protein by binding nitrogen and carbon through biological transmutation within the body. Some waters are more alive than others. Water that has a high percentage of quartz crystal colloids helps maintain and restore vitality. It serves as a catalyst in transmitting the morphogenic field that is present.

Once a circle, such as a morphogenic field, is created, it becomes self-sustaining on the level of superconduction, which is held in a delicate temperature niche because of resonance. You can witness this in nature in the healthy growth of a plant that grows inside a circle of stones. What is the force in life that allows you to defy gravity and levitate? We can lift the weight of an object up and off the earth effortlessly with the help of magnetic fields, the same way two opposite poles of a magnet work.

Nature's force field is projected out of a vortex, which manifests itself as spinning electrons, and the transformation that this energy expresses. Thought has been shown to influence the growth of seedlings and the mind has been proven capable of bending metals and interacting on an electronic and mechanical level. An upset person may experience many more computer crashes than a contented person. Happy thoughts create an alkaline field and bitterness causes the battery to go flat. One good example of this that has stumped physicians for years is the fact that people's wrist watches die when they pass on. It is such a common occurrence that it is often noted in medical reports, almost as an afterthought.

Angstrom-sized bismuth[45] transmits feeling, sound, and sight and acts as a wave-guide. A living body is composed of electrons in perpetual motion. Life is composed of a blueprint that morphogenically causes the assemblage and manifestation of elements operating on the level of neutrinos and electrons through biological transmutation. Algae and moss can grow in midair, hanging by a wire. Aerobic bacteria and minerals are created by stirring colloidal quartz crystal in purified filtered water, just like we do in our highly alkaline-charged water (see recipe in Appendix).

However, the body makes use of random energy fluctuations. The body has an innate intelligence that thermogenically regulates the temperature within a narrow margin that supports the body's maximum vitality.

Life is aglow with electrons that have unusual behaviors. In monatomic elements, electrons pair up and are under a protective, orderly screening. Zero-point energetics arises naturally as the sink and the power source are in synchronicity. Residuum wave energetics emit a transform from this space that acts like a vacuum on a micro-scale.

The ethmoid organ, tuned to lines of geomagnetic polar force, has the largest amount of natural load stone crystals in the body. It picks up geomagnetic micropulsations coming off the surface of the Earth that naturally set the circadian and ultradian cycles of the body. Ancient Chinese medicine teaches us about these cycles, such as the gallbladder meridian hour that occurs at 3 P.M. and in turn stimulates glycogen output from the liver later that night at 3 A.M. The electrogravitic force fields of electrons flow from negative toward positive.

Today's Healers

Medical doctors who become highly specialized in one area remark that it is challenging for them to understand cross-disciplinary insight. Typically, conversation is restricted to the agreed upon understanding of technical concepts that licensed practitioners of medicine are taught to believe. Many are twentieth-century fit, yet, this we are living in the twenty-first century. Many doctors are comfortable where they are. It is interesting to note a study in which first year medical students reported that they felt nutrition to be one of the most important aspects for healing and good health. Eight years later this group was questioned again, now as interns, and respond that there is very little relationship between nutrition and healing disease. Their new mode of thinking is that drugs and surgery are the best approaches to healing. Quite a lot of classic brainwashing techniques are enlisted to change the students' minds to achieve this end. These techniques include sleep deprivation and bombarding students with massive client loads while interning (some thirty-five patients a day is common). One oral surgeon intern flatly told me, "I used to care, Annie, but now I just slap a prescription on them or schedule a surgery as fast as I can and get them out of there. I don't have time to care anymore." He said it was common for him to be scheduled for thirty to forty patients during his internship, and by the end of it the healer within was slain and the drug-pusher and knife-wielder was out front and in charge. It is only in medicine that we find this rigorous brainwashing. We don't find it in any other field. Can you imagine an art student that had to bang out thirty paintings a day, or the lawyer who had to defend thirty cases a day? I know many disenchanted medical students who left school when they could see that their dream of becoming a great healer couldn't be realized within allopathic medicine, that the art of healing had been lost.

Medicine used to be referred to as the healing arts; we have always understood that there is an art to healing. Any time someone has comforted you and relieved you of pain, any parent that lays a caring hand over their child's forehead, you can remember that healing is a God-given birthright—the right to be healed and to heal others. Each of us has this potential, and some healers are especially gifted. The art of healing needs to be returned to the healing arts.

Zero Point and Vacuum Polarization

Zero point is where two equal and opposite waves cancel each other out. Zero point causes vacuum. What is left over is called a residuum vibration. This vibration is a reflection of vitality. This very fine vibration, you could say, is a resonance that is monopolar and creates a chain reaction that keeps electrons in a perpetual continuous flow (superconduction).

As time-forward and time-reverse electrons pair up, matter becomes pure energy. It may seem that where there exists nothing, not even a space that's considered a particle, that the space was squeezed to nothing. Yet, there is a fluctuating electric field in this empty space. We will keep things light here as far as quantum gravitics and zero-point energetics is concerned. Maybe you remember being small and a parent or friend throwing you up high in the air and catching you. The point where you reached very top, before falling back down again, there was a feeling of floating and a flutter as your stomach and heart met. You learned to contract the tummy slightly to control the unpleasant stimulus. Mastery over that sensation gives us a feeling of euphoria. We learn to override the unpleasant feeling to come to really enjoy the experience.

Electrons are most often out of groove, causing matter to emit a slight wobble that gives all matter a personal signature. Our constitution is this vibration. This includes how well our learned behavior enables mastery in any given moment. Either you have a good amplitude of electricity to give you generous access to both sides of the brain and the frontal cortex, or you operate from limited brain function that exhibits a low amplitude of electricity.

A monopolar light is emitted as sink and source are in resonance, which causes electrons to line up. This functions in much the same manner as when you have two violins in a room that are both similarly tuned, when the E string on one violin is plucked and it causes the E string on the other violin to resonate sympathetically. This resonance is what turns up the amplitude of electricity in the body.

Fragrance, taste, and attraction are examples of sensing deeply subatomic properties. On this plane, the elementary particles we are composed of are organized transforms (spatial resonance) in a sea of zero-point energy. The fluctuations or residuum vibration are the same. There is a vacuum created by the joining of positive and negative electrons, which become one as pure light. Neutrino mass and electron spin involve unique vacuum zero-point energy to arise as a residuum vibration. The charge of electrons flows from positive to negative. Our ethereal body is really the vacuum polarization of an electron conduction cloud. These collapsing electrons stabilize in turn into a standing wave[46] within us. There is a vacuum polarization in the biological transmutation of electrons where we find imploding protons, nucleons, and heavy ions that then cause a standing wave to arise that is quite symmetrical rather than globular. Organic matter is created in this vacuum polarization of negatively charged electrons.

Displacement currents flow from symmetrical and round lines of force to interact with each other. Vacuum polarization is powerfully synergistic when more than one ion or nucleus is involved in the plasma of our body. Ion acoustic oscillations arise as waves of vacuum polarization displacement currents. The more orderliness within the system the more intense the vacuum polarization effect that lithes our whole body by strengthening the amplitude of the flowing electrons. Enjoying a sweetness of life causes the ions in our plasma body to synchronistically oscillate together. Ion acoustic activity is sound made luminous.

Ball lightning coming out of the ground in a storm is akin to what happens energetically inside the body of a person who is having a nervous breakthrough (a reframe for nervous breakdown), where 180-degree turns in the ion acoustic wave pattern enfold upon itself to form a ring. Biological transmutation involves unique particle interactions in polarization of the vacuum. Ions and conductive electrons each have unique radiation patterns. How fast or slow a person's pace and ease of moving is can generate great inner light or shut down this light quite dramatically, respectively.

Particle spin of an electron during its perpetual motion is shaped by zero-point energetics. As long as there is excellent overall body pH, electrons will flow in an orderly way without much change or eddy current losses, resulting in a high degree of order. There is a smooth flow rather than a magnetic drag as ionization takes place. If switching polarity takes place in our plasma, radiation can double in the body. Magnetic poles can completely reverse, showing that it really is a property of the ether (negative time energy).

Muscle movement takes place because of the body's use of the ether/ gravity forces of attraction and repulsion. The background pH maintains the balance of forces that allow chemical reactions to take place. The pH in our body is like a painter's canvas. The body does not possess its own intrinsic energy on its own. The body has a physical nature we can feel; but our light body possesses an energy that it receives directly from the environment.

Natural observations with magnets have led scientists to conclude that magnetism polarity is a property of ether. Previous thought was that magnetism was simply a property owned by a stone. The physical body is anchored, and yet, the mind traverses time and space. Time simply flows through the body and all that is physical. Time is suspended in the present as the future is drawn ever into this moment. The present moment has the future moving toward it, while the past has a trace of the present.

Plasma of ether flows through the body and through all things; in fact, it is the very fundamental energy that animates the universe. Vacuum energetics and zero-point energy either produce or annihilate electrons. The space we occupy, which consists of the physical material that composes us, has a physical attributes that involves the rotating of electrons orbiting a mass of nucleons and positrons that are being moved around inside us. In turn, this movement is moved by the Earth and then pulled by the sun, which itself orbits the galaxy—all in perpetual motion. The inner world of the body (microcosm) reflects the great outer world (macrocosm).

Universal lines of intelligence are woven into the very fabric of the space we occupy. Matter is created and annihilated from our physical space in a continuous cycle. Strange attractors are constantly being assembled, projected into the future that is bearing down on us in our present moment. It is this arrangement of space inside of us that gives us an external form. Nature is the perfect expression of space energy in the generation of matter. There are hot and cold forms of energy, such as black tar pavement and cool green grass in the summer, demonstrating an astronomical temperature difference in the same season. Rocks and other material placed in the same room can have different temperatures.

As humans, we are only in tune to the smallest piece of the electromagnetic spectrum; other creatures, however, rely on this spectrum for their very existence and can exhibit a greater awareness of such things. The brain of the dolphin and porpoise evolved 30 million years ago! They are the only other creatures that have as many, or more, high-energy electrons around the brain as we do—and they have very high globulin levels, indicating great intelligence. They have much larger cerebral cortexes than humans, suggesting a multileveled and evolved language system that we are only just beginning to decipher.

Nature's tendency is to form circles. Thus, cells are excellent resonators, emitting and absorbing radiation. Blood emits and absorbs radiation of the highest frequency in the body. Life is a symphony of sequential multiple radiators. Resonance is happening as cells and life colloids are radiating together, one upon the other. Disease manifests itself out of a desperate need for cell oscillatory equilibrium and harmony inside. On the healthy/growing side of the bell curve, cellular radiation lights up your whole body, while on the decomposing side nature recycles through the growth of mold, fungus, yeast, and other pleomorphic organisms that have grown unchecked by very low cell resonance.

We maintain good vitality by practicing LifeFood habits and avoiding the consumption of inert dead material. The finer vibrations within the body carry the larger ones. Maintaining vital cell vibration is the key to reversing disease. Cell nuclei are electrical oscillating circuits. DNA filaments within the nuclei oscillate according to a specific frequency.

Space is bent in on itself in specific ways which modify cosmic radiation. Far infrared[47] radiation heats us up. Cells and life possess a sink that enables a direct tapping into cosmic radiation, allowing us to oscillate according to a specific natural frequency. Cells, in the order of 200 quintillion, all vibrate with their own personal signature. In health this happens in harmony.

How To Access Universal Energy

The universe is alive with energy; vibrating energy permeates everything. The fig still on the vine is receives life force. Upon being picked the life force being transmitted from the fig tree is abruptly cut. The fruit, from this moment on, is warmed to ripeness by the heat of the sun.

Energy and vibration are everything in the universe. All known elements have a unique vibration. Carbon and iron each have specific rates of vibration. Colloids from a fruit or a rushing mountain stream have very different properties from mined salts found in dried-up inland desert lakes. Living elements within the body are drawn into enlightenment and strive to be in tune with universal energy.

Vitality ensues as organs like the thyroid gland ionize elements in the body plasma. The thyroid gland creates a field of energy, as do the hippocampus, pineal, and other glands. Like a well-organized friction grid that causes space to conform, the thyroid ionizes substance that act as information for distant cells.

Life colloids are always in motion and operate as transceivers. Cells exposed to lower-end electromagnetics (broadcast band) drink in electrons at their resonance frequency. Cells drink electrons in until they are brimming. Once the current is flowing nothing else can be added. Surprisingly little is taught about these subjects in medical school. Healing does involve electro-magno-gravitic forces. Being in resonance greatly speeds up the healing process. Medical schools could delve deeper into the factors that create health, rather than disease.

Upstream Preventative Medicine

To help a less than healthy river or stream eliminate pollution one has to start at the source of contamination. If the plumbing were leaking, it would be useless to try to sweep the floor. One has to apply common sense and create a list of priorities. LifeFood Nutrition and the body's colloidal health is essentially preventative medicine that involves upstream treatment.

LifeFood Nutrition, electric herbs, and charged alkaline water contribute to preventative medicine. People have made the mistake of focusing attention on what is in the food rather than how the food is metabolized within the digestive tract. For instance, flesh putrefies and metabolizes into amines; vegetables grown with artificial fertilizers metabolize into nitrates. The combining of amines and nitrates will form highly carcinogenic nitrosamines. Stinky bowel movements result from putrefaction and fermentation in the digestive tract. Drinking charged alkaline water and eating a clean diet of LifeFood greatly assists intestinal hygiene, reducing indoles, skatols, phenols, histamines, ammonia, and hydrogen sulfide that help obtain sweeter-smelling defecation, a reflection of cleaner stools.

Alkaline Water Is Superior to Antioxidants

Alkaline water and LifeFood contribute significantly to feeling better and thinking more clearly. While we need alkaline water and LifeFood colloids internally, slightly acidic water is generally best for bathing as it acts as an antiseptic for the skin. Alkaline water has a high negative redox potential which quickly permeates the cells and body fluids, decreasing the oxidization (aging) of the body by donating its abundant electrons to free radical oxygen molecules. This produces an excess of electrons to donate to peroxide and hydroxel radicals. Blood built of LifeFood colloids has a negative charge and the proper anionic alkaline valence (electrical energy field). Body fluids charged by colloids with a large negative redox potential are highly structured, have smaller molecules in atomic shells, and have highly absorbent molecular bonds.

Spare Electrons Equal Downstream Cell Protection

Alkaline colloidal nutrition enters the liver, lymph, and organs quickly because of its low molecular weight and its smaller particle cluster size. Alkaline colloids, with their safe redox (oxidation reduction) potential, donate electrons freely to neutralize active oxygen. Normal cells acquire the electrons needed to grow, mature, regenerate, and function from cosmic energy that is condensed during the night.

Colloidal particles have an enormous surface area and possess a negative electrical charge. The smaller the colloid the greater its ability to hold its charge. Colloids of life can derive their electron transfer energy from fermentation if they are without oxygen. Cells, viral-like particles (spores), microorganisms, yeasts, and pleomorphic life forms made of dysbiotic life colloids all get their energy from fermentation, and they secrete all kinds of mycotoxic acid wastes.

All Beings Are Ferments Given Certain Conditions

Fermentation occurs at our very substrate. We start out as simple fetal endoblastic cells. From fertilization until the sixth week of embryonic life, our cells predominantly draw energy through fermentation. All organisms possess within them conditions that cause the availability of oxygen to be momentarily suspended.

An egg contains simple colloids and initially lacks organization. If the egg is shaken vigorously, its sugar and glycogen disappear and you find alcohol, acetic acid, and butyric acid in their place. Fermentation has taken place. This is the work of "life colloids" acting as ferments. The colloids of cells live beyond the life of the being and organ that they are a part of. The minerals of these colloids may be found incorporated into all the histological elements of the body and can be recovered as living colloids from the soil after death. When further introduced into a culture, there is a characteristic "life colloid" that has the potential to express itself within that cellular medium again.

Just as light draws a curved path through the ethos, colloids of life hold evolved elliptical asymmetrical patterns within themselves. From the elliptical asymmetrical carbon patterns of growth, to life colloids, to bacteria-like spirochete, pallid and numerous other spiral movements arise from the spinning asymmetry of colloids that compose the body.

Colloids of life (from the monera of the food eaten) join to make strings that circle and fold back in on themselves during the passage of the digestive tract, forming resonance circles, then bubbles (red blood cells), as they wash down the coastline of the intestinal villi. During fasting, blood forms first from fat cells while blood sugar is still available; otherwise, the protein of our body, muscle tissue, can be transformed into blood. These colloids of life are transported throughout the body as blood.

Most people are born healthy, yet, over time we can become challenged by poor diet, negative emotions, and/or injury. Intestinal flora becomes compromised by drugs and antibiotics in an oxygen-starved environment. Bacteria, fungus, and yeast can build up inside the body. As we age we may feel the effects of not having kept our alkalinity and aerobic self from becoming acidic and anaerobic (without oxygen). Then fungus, mold, yeast, and bacteria in this state feed off glucose, nucleic acids, and lipids and excrete mycotoxic waste products. The terrain of the body becomes unkempt. In this situation, growth of pleomorphic life colloids rises up progressively and pushes deeper into the body.

When adequate oxygen is unavailable, the very colloids we are made of become assembled into unfriendly life colloids that produce hundreds of toxins. These unpleasant life colloids metabolize sugar to produce acetaldehyde, ethyl alcohol, and methane gas.

Life begets life and death begets death. Acid-forming and catarrh-forming foods bury us. It's like digging your own grave with your spoon. Even vegetarians on a macrobiotic diet who eat cooked grains as half of their daily intake can often have out-of-control blood sugar. Vegetarian junk food is abundant. Mold- and fungus-forming foods like cake, bread, pasta, rice, wheat, potatoes, soy or rice milk, and pasteurized fruit juice create addictions. They are drugs! A single can of soda contains about nine teaspoons of sugar. Many fit right into either an opiate or stimulant receptor in the brain. The body is only designed to put together the amino acids it has as information molecules (polypeptides) or nutrient carriers (chelates).

Life colloids (spores, bacteria, molds, fungus, yeasts, phytoplankton) change their form as the terrain of the body changes. Modern medicine has taught a less than truthful doctrine called "monomorphism" that proclaims that disease is caused by external, unchanging monomorphic (one-form) microbes that invade the body. They stand by their belief that this invader should be cut, burned, and poisoned. Unfortunately, this behavior results in fungus-derived mycotoxins. These mycotoxin-seeded spores are responsible for pneumonia, candida, and many ear conditions. Common colloidal life forms like bacteria have evolved into super strains, now deemed "untreatable" by all known chemical means, including antibiotics. Simple immune challenges have now become major health challenges because of antibiotic abuse. It is extremely easy to catch pneumonia or staff infection in the hospital these days, even though you come in for something else entirely. In fact, drug- and surgery-based hospital care is listed as the number three cause of death in America. A patient goes in for a gallbladder-removal operation and dies a few days later of a staph infection; or, a patient goes in for a liver biopsy and later dies of a heart attack. My uncle checked to the hospital for his leukemia and died there of pneumonia a week later. He didn't die of his disease; he died of the treatment methods prescribed.

During live blood cell analysis, or phase contrast and dark field live cell microscopy, we see life colloids (pleomorphic organisms) change their form. We see aggregates of colloids from blood cells and the body serum fusing into spicules; spores fusing together to move and wiggle to become bacteria; and bacteria collecting into a mass of mold, fungal, or yeast forms. We have seen these life colloids assembling themselves from blood plasma, from undigested proteins, from starches of cooked denatured food, and from poorly formed red blood cells.

Friendly life colloids live in saphritic relationship with us. They build us and help our cell respiration. Fibrin and platelets, for aiding in cell repair and blood clotting, are "life colloids." They can change into colloids that wiggle and have a bubble body shape, or sometimes a rod shape. Sometimes they assemble themselves into an acid-fast, cell-wall deficient unfriendly colloid like bacteria.

The key to health is a boosted immune system. When we heat colloids we find that they once again become ferments. Boiled fruit juice is a sterile fluid that will go on to become turbid. This is less than excellent nutrition.

Life colloids like ferments, bacteria, and yeasts live without oxygen and secrete toxic byproducts. The ancient Egyptians' embalming techniques included removing the mycotoxic gut and brain to help preserve the deceased's form. Under the live blood cell microscope, we watch a white snow substance become a virtual hail that fuzzes out the light as L-form bacteria proliferate unchecked. The goodness of an apple is gone when mold appears on any part of it, so dump it in the compost rather than trying to salvage any of it. The mold simply metastasizes. Mold that you can see on the surface of that jar of jam signifies that the mold has permeated the entire jarful.

While the body has oxygen, symbiotic life colloids ensure health. At other times, dysbiotic life colloids grow out of our substrate material, attaching themselves and creating cross-linkages between our cells. These fermentative life colloids assemble themselves onto organs, blood cells, and intracellular and extracellular fluids. They excrete all kinds of toxins. Bacteria excrete lactic acids! Fungus excretes acetaldehyde and uric acid, a toxin that reduces to ethanol and then to formaldehyde in the liver—the hangover toxin. Some people act quite drunk on a starch- and sugar-based denatured diet.

Blood Alkalinity, Tachyons, and Energy

Body alkalinity supports health. Blood alkalinity is the effect of ions in solution (electrolytes) or colloids' energy field (scalar wave) stemming from electrons, spinning ever so gently to the left around their nuclei. Anions and cations ionize when they come together and energy is given off. Anions spiral counterclockwise, up toward the sky and the Van Allen Belts on the outside of the ionosphere surrounding the Earth; whereas cations spiral clockwise, down toward the center of the earth. Colloids require anionic energy. Minerals drawn in through food are either anionic or cationic—limes or carrots, respectively. An element's counterclockwise spinning energy field creates a grid of resistance. Tachyons passing through this grid precipitate into electrons.

Imagine a subatomic particle of unknown mass traveling faster than light. Tachyon energetics is responsible for behaviors such as attraction, fragrance, taste, and feelings. It is theorized that tachyons are what free energy machines draw energy from. Wherever there is gravity tachyon energy is found. Everything is composed of cosmic energy that condenses, precipitating into tachyons. Tachyons then condense to precipitate into electrons. The magnetic charge every cell receives in an alkaline body converts tachyon energy into biologically usable electrons.

Tachyons are converted into electrons when the cells have the correct potassium/sodium relationship. An abundance of sodium in relationship to potassium would short out this process of converting free energy (tachyons) into electrons. This supraluminal (beyond light) energy is creating order. Complementary particles, even light years apart, change polarities simultaneously as tachyons fly from one complementary particle to the other and change their spins.

Blood is 70 percent water and 30 percent colloids. Blood is supposed to have a pH of about 7.3,[48] whereas body cells have an internal pH of about 6.8, except for the nucleus of the cell and the stomach acid. In order to quench free-radical activity and neutralize hydroxyl radicals, the body serum has to be alkaline. It uses electrons to neutralize acids like free-radical peroxidase into water and oxygen. Our body fluids must have a negative electrical voltage to keep things dissolved in the blood and body serum, to sweep them along to the liver. Alkalinity dissolves the crystals of acid within the body that form in a toxic medium.

Robust vitality requires an alkaline body to draw energy from oxidation. Flashlight batteries have electricity while they are alkaline, but lose their electricity the moment they become acidic. Our body functions much like a wet cell battery. Because most food people eat is cationic, digestive fluids need to be anionic. The dance of life involves these minute minerals having the proper electrical charge in relationship to each other.

Colloids of Life Change Shape

Colloids from food are assembled into and become incorporated as red blood cells (erythrocytes), body cells, and some sixteen unique microorganisms. Our blood-clotting factor is actually an organism! Colloids of life stream from (as if growing out of) the substrate of devitalized red blood cells, then pool to become a monera (a swarming pool of life colloids), out of which can spring nucleated somatic cells, leucocytes, lymphatic, or other endothelial cells, as well as bacteria, molds, fungi, or other pleomorphic life.

Symbiotic or dysbiotic organisms arise from the our substrate if the terrain allows. The terrain of these colloids of life determines the type of life form they are fashioned into. This is nature's way of renewing body cells and recycling the spent structure along with all else that has lived to return it back into space dust.

Monomorphism is a false doctrine taught where a life colloid (bacteria, yeast, mold or fungus) has only one form. One can conclude from present microscopy that:

- the life colloid is endowed with pleomorphism (many changing forms).

- pleomorphic development is controlled by blood borne inhibitors.

- growth hormone is generated by the life colloid's cycle. In the animal and plant world, cellular division requires primitive colloids of life (life colloid, spore and double spore).

- when blood borne inhibitors are lacking, growth hormone is allowed to increase to the point where it compromises cellular metabolism and stimulated cellular growth.

COLLOIDS OF LIFE IN A HEALTHY BODY transform into life colloids, then spores; spores then transmutate into double spores. These three pleomorphic organisms—life colloid, spore, and double spore—produce important life substances (including growth hormone) and perform other functions that support life. They are also necessary constituents of healthy blood.

Primitive pleomorphic organisms help to program the cells absorption of enzymes, minerals, vitamins, and other nutrients. Colloids from simple life colloids like phytoplankton or soil-born microbes become easily incorporated into the body as they are quickly assimilated into every conceivable aspect of our physical structure and bodily function. These colloids help bring about a balance of anions and cations so our terrain (body pH) is kept intact.

Environments too alkaline or acidic allow pleomorphic organisms like spores, double spores, bacteria, mold, fungus, and yeast to arise. The condition that allows fungus to arise is cancer's endpoint. The body must maintain a balance of friendly and unfriendly life colloids.

False Doctrine of Orthodox Theory on Blood Formation

To recap, the orthodox theory believes that:
1) blood cells originate through cell division by mitosis,
2) red blood cells are highly differentiated and incapable of differentiating into any other cells,
3) red blood cells simply degenerate after carrying oxygen and carbon dioxide,
4) blood cells cannot pass through capillaries and the thin layer of endothelial cells.

Colloidal Biology, Blood, and Cells

Colloids make up erythroblast or mesenchymal elements in the connective tissue, blood vessels, blood, the entire lymphatic system, heart, and portions of the mesoderm. The colloids assemble themselves into bubbles (erythrocytes) as a result of aggregates forming and then fusing together. Cells arise out of living substances where there aren't any nucleated cells. We see this everywhere in nature—in the protein substance inside an egg, or as in the body from the colloidal protoplasm of the blood corpuscle.

With a special dark field microscope we can witness and document colloids of the cytoplasm of red blood cells extruding and streaming out to join with colloids of the body serum and the extrusion of other red blood cells to form a monera (colloidal mass). Symbiotic and dysbiotic simple life colloids, depending on the terrain (somatic cell or white blood cell, spores, bacteria, mold, fungus, and yeast), arise out of the monera of these pooled colloids.

Under fasting conditions, fat cells and all extraneous material is disassembled and discarded or reassembled into healthy cell architecture. As we fast the fat of our body becomes the colloids that in turn become blood.

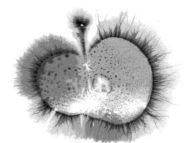

CHAPTER 10

Cell Rejuvenation

Keys To Solving Cancer

In clarifying the origin of cancer cells, it's important to note that the colloids of cancer originate from red blood cells. The current orthodox view is that cancer cells originate from epithelial cells—a mutation increased through mitotic cell division. The view presented in colloidal biology is that red blood cells differentiate into cancer cells in pathological terrain and conditions of the body. It has long been known that spores, (viruses), bacteria, and other simple colloids of life arise spontaneously in degenerating protoplasm. Cancer spores (acid-fast cell-wall deficient bacteria) are the result of degenerated red blood cells. Cancer is a chronic general disease rather than a local condition, which is the presently held and favored orthodox view.

Healing requires that the blood become normal. Prevention should always be first. Allopathic treatment (typical hospital care) is missing a fundamental healing therapeutic. A reduction in diet superlatively quickens healing. A blood bandage quickens healing. The colloids of the red blood actually become connective tissue. The colloids of stagnated red blood cells can tax the spleen and liver and cause them to hypertrophy. Healing involves normalizing erythrocyte poiesis in the intestinal villi and cleaning from the top of the mountain for the lymph, which is the area surrounding the liver, gallbladder, pancreas, stomach, heart, and intestine.

Lengthen Your Lifespan

Most people would be surprised to learn of an ancient health practice termed urine therapy—the practice of drinking a few ounces of one's own fresh urine as a tonic for its rich content of hormones, antibodies, and many nutrients and agents that combat infection and mold, fungus, and yeast. You may be surprised to realize that you've already practiced this. Urea, usually gathered commercially from animals and also other sources, is added to most skin/hair softening lotions and conditioners. Urea is the most potent agent on the planet for softening the skin and hair. For the last thirty years in America the most prescribed medication has been Premarin, pregnant mare urine; it is the hormone-replacement therapy derived from the urine of a pregnant mare that millions of women the world over take on a daily basis. Urine is really purified blood minus the pigment, rather than a waste product as some might assume. The waste of the body exits through the intestine as fecal debris.

Urine therapy, taking a few ounces of one's own fresh urine, caught midstream on the morning's first pee, works in a similar fashion to enriching your soil through composting. Let's take a closer look at urine. What's in it? Urine is a saline solution that contains many colloidal vitamins and minerals; it is loaded with your own hormones and when it's the first catch of the day it's rich with your own human growth hormone (HGH), which is secreted from your brain during the darkest hours of the night while you sleep. Perhaps urine's most alluring feature is the abundance of coded antibodies to any tagged toxins you have come in contact with during the previous few days. In other words, it's your own perfect autogenic vaccine with your exact coding of hormones and antibodies because you produced them. Science could never produce such a match. The only real rule with urine therapy is to avoid taking pharmaceutical drugs, including pharmaceutical-grade vitamin/mineral supplements, which include all supplements unless they are whole food vitamin/mineral complexes.

Bringing in your own fresh urine increases tissue and body fluid content of urea. Urea has an intimate relationship with albumin. Albumin is the super-protein transporter in the blood and a high level of albumin indicate high intelligence, excellent health and immunity. Uric acid balance is a component of the body's chemical-mediated immunity. Administering uric acid can help keep people alive in the last chronic stages of life because of these immune effects and the fact that it is bacteriostatic.

Urea and silica also are polar-constructed hydrotropic materials that help promote proper hydration of the connective tissue of the body; otherwise, the cells inside shrink. When cells shrink they are aging. This reduction inside the cell surface results in compromised cell processes, like enzyme functioning.

Urea and uric acid in urine is amazing in its bacteriostatic effects. It's one of the few organic substances that can neutralize polio and has wonderful tuberculostatic effect. The higher the concentrations of urea the more efficient the bacteriostatic effect that clears the body of toxins. Excessive drinking of acid-forming beverages, and even acidic water, cause us to lose precious stores of uric acid. Urea can completely alter the shape of microorganisms, as can the lactic acid of fresh fruits and vegetables. It helps wounds heal and helps dissolve spent protein.

The protein-solvent properties of uric acid and urea have caused it to be effectively used to treat many pathogenic conditions. Urine improves blood flow and lymph circulation. It allows leukocytic activity to continue uninterrupted. It has polypeptides, which show enormous virulence against the most pathogenic bacteria, and urea has been administered in emergencies to revive people from prophylactic shock.

Urine is a cache of nutrients including natural DHEA, interleukin, urokinase, and antigen-specific growth factors. It has protein globulins and immunoglobulins and gastric secretory depressant. Uric acid controls free radicals and urine has other anti-cancer substances like antineoplastons, H-11, beta-indol acetic acid, directin, three methyl gly-oxal, allatoin, factor s, and protease. Your daily cache of urine includes glycine, glutamic acid, cystine, Vitamin C, allanine, arginine, lysine, pantothenic acid, and Vitamin B6.

The curative effects of urea comes about because the positively charged protein of the body's plasma binds with the negative charge of the colloid. (This is rare to find except in silica.) This causes opalescence phenomenon (scattering of light particles the size of 300 to 5,000 angstroms; a hydrogen atom is 1-angstrom wide). Without hydrotropic materials of the blood along with proper levels of albumin, body hydration drops and blood flocculation and coagulation can occur.

Plasma proteins are amphoretic, meaning they combine with either an acid or an alkaline base. However, albumins coagulate with heat. Blood plasma proteins, albumin in particular, make up roughly 75 percent of the total plasma proteins in a healthy person and transport most of the colloids that become incorporated into the cells of our body. Albumin brings moisture into the connective tissue, moisturizing us in our entirety. Starvation and aging is the process of reduction of plasma proteins of the body fluids.

Rejuvenation equals optimizing hydration of albumin in the body. Colloidal albumin helps dissolve fat, lipid, and esters in water; sodium makes this possible. LifeFood protein colloids are hydrophilic (water-attracting). They are found near the surface of the molecule. Those elements that are more hydrophobic (water-repelling) are found near the interior of the molecule, away from solvency.

Silica, like in the herb horsetail, and fresh urine contain hydrotropic elements that facilitate proper hydration and softening of connective tissues, preventing shrinkage. Silica is amazing in that it binds temporarily with nitrogen, which then binds with carbon; as soon as the protein material begins to form, silicon splits away. Silicon is integral in the formation of protein and life itself.

Diatoms are single-celled organisms that use fat, volutin,[49] and photosynthesis to supply their energy needs. Diatoms occupy about 5,000 species of algae and supply up to 70 percent of the Earth's oxygen! When they give their bodies up they give up a cache of colloidal silica. This is diatomaceous earth. The decay of diatoms involves a polymerization of silica from the skeleton of the diatom and as a result of this process an oxygen molecule is released into the atmosphere. Only after the decay of the diatom began on Earth was energy able to be used as oxygen. Certain enzymes are needed to convert oxygen to energy. Energy that comes from the use of oxygen in metabolism of sugar can be fifteen times stronger with the phosphoralisation of ATP through fermentation. Also, without silica, protein synthesis ceases and fat metabolism is compromised. In this case, cells fatten, revealing an oxygen use disturbance/starvation. Silica plays a major role in cancer therapy.

Where there is less light silica assumes the metabolic process. Silica-rich foods include asparagus, cauliflower, horseradish, lettuce, millet, and sunflower. Herbals that contain colloids of silica help bind to proteins, making them miscible in the body fluid. Urea and silica help stimulate cell metabolism. The mucopolysaccharide packing material around the cells helps keep a constant streaming of electrons into the cell while it draws water, and other cellular waste out. This important process occurs through maintaining the proper level of polar-constructed hydrotropic materials, which urea and silica provide.

Just to give you an idea of the size of things we are talking about here, an angstrom is the diameter of a hydrogen atom and is 10^8cm. Colloids range from 10 to 10,000 angstroms! Colloids are not true solutions like sugar and salt. These sugar and salt particles are smaller and composed of only a few atoms.

When colloidal particles do connect, they like to join with strings that coil and make up a colloidal protein in a living substance. While there are spare electrons in this colloidal material, this joining causes a scattering of light and a field of energy that keep them apart from each other. Colloidal particles are small enough to resist and are unaffected by gravity.

The solid particle of a colloid is called a sol. There are two types of colloidal particle dispersions depending on whether the particles are occurring in a liquid, solid, or a gas. Gaseous elements cannot exist as colloids. Only the solid mineral elements act as a colloid medium.

The most important element of our blood plasma is its colloidal protein integrity. The two types of sols can be divided into two subgroups: 1) molecular sols: single giant molecules dispersed in liquid. These include most organic sols. 2) micellar sols: aggregates of smaller atoms, ions, and molecules dispersed in a liquid.

Colloids are in a perpetual state of motion due to the spare electrons they posses. The molecules of room temperature water are traveling at about 14,000 miles per hour. This is happening around each molecule, which means that we are without any net movement.

Ingestion of heat-processed protein denatures and soils the body. Colloidal protein is made up of a coil. This very tight coil of minerals and other elements are strung together in a tiny spherical ball. When we heat protein it causes these coils to unwind and the protein becomes viscous. The colloid particles are held together by weak bonds that break, causing some of the colloids to become ionically bound to each other; others break as the protein is heated and becomes more hydrophobic. The cooking and denaturing of protein causes a viscosity and the bonding of the colloids to become ionically bound (rather than covalently bound) making the molecule semi-solid.

If we took one gram of colloidal silica in its LifeFood state and we put each colloid next to each other, it would make up an area of more than 300 square yards! If you took one cubic inch of the LifeFood colloids and put their surface area in their uncooked state next to each other, it would make up more than 50,000 square feet.

If you took the colloids of one cubic inch of silica and you lined up the particles, end to end in a straight line, the particles would stretch the distance seventeen times to the moon and back! This surface area causes an enormous activation and ability for protein synthesis to occur in the body. The effect of cooking these colloids has the same effect as shortening this distance (thus effect) of the colloids to equal a distance of seventeen times from Houston to New York and back rather than to the moon.

Purifying the Lymph at the Top of the Mountain

That area of our body where the small intestine draws colloids from lipids (smaller than a wave length of light) is in through the lacteals ducts and Peyer's patches of lymph nodes. Colloids in lipids become miscible as they are bound to protein carriers. A poor diet and sedentary lifestyle affect the lymphatics, causing this important system that drains any molecules larger than can fit in the blood vessels to slow and become stagnant.

Adhesions of fibrin and globulin, denatured particles like tars and resins, can limit the ability for absorption of bile back into the body. These adhesions emanate from the gallbladder to the small intestine and from the gallbladder to the stomach, pancreas, heart, and colon and can inhibit passage of the metabolites needed in the body for ensuring we have a good connection between the autonomic nervous system and the proteins in the body serum that make up the cerebral spinal fluid in the brain.

Only one in 230 particles of albumin are small enough to make it into the brain. These are High Density Lipoproteins (HDLs). These raw materials flow with electrons that stimulate the flow of lymphatic system and to come in through the area of the body involving the gallbladder. This area has to be working well for a person's lymphatic system to function. Diet and lifestyle deeply influence this function, and the lymphatic system is compromised more than any other system when it is not working properly.

The top of the mountain in our body is the area around the gallbladder where lipids and proteins combine. This area can have an enormous outpouring of alkaline salts because of lavish eating. The area around the gallbladder has direct connections through lymphatic and connective tissue to the stomach, heart, pancreas, colon, and lungs and can create a source of irritation to these vital organs when things aren't going well.

The integrity of the lacteals ducts and Peyer's patches from the small intestine to the gallbladder itself reveal the vitality of the person. This absorption area is an important element in the etiology of most physical conditions—more than any other single condition, for the most part.

The liver is always compromised when health challenges arise. The colloids coming from castor oil can help bring raw materials in a form that electrifies the top of the mountain where lymph is produced in the body. Castor oil is a biochemist's delight. Castor oil has been called "the palm of Christ" for its amazing healing properties from its rich cache of medicinal colloids. Castor oil is incredibly stable and possesses unique properties that allow it to be incorporated into many chemical reactions. We insist that castor packs (poultice) be administered over the liver area during the 14-Day LifeFood Nutritional Fast. It really is a miracle worker in the way it softens adhesions and loosens tars, wax, and resins that have been stored for decades in tired organs and in the abdominal cavity. Three castor packs a day during the fast can potentiate your cleanse by 50 percent!

Blood Factors Maintain Vital Immunity

Barometric pressure and sunspot activity produce physical phenomena that tune the body senses to read the environment like a barometer and sundial do. Long ago, when oxygen was less available in the atmosphere, moisture displaced oxygen. Thus, low barometric pressure allowed less oxygen within the body. During this time, life colloids were disassembled and reassembled into life forms that could draw energy from fermentation.

The immune system relies on friendly life colloids to keep unfriendly ones at bay. Antibiotic drugs are grossly abused in this country, which displays an ignorance of our evolutionary process. L. Salivarius, cultured from human breast milk colostrums, is a friendly bacterium that disassembles unfriendly life colloids. We are supposed to get our life's supply of colostrum in the first few days of life from our mother's breast. We then begin colonizing L. Salivarius in the small and large intestines. It's interesting to note that the bacterium known as vancomycin-resistant enteroccus, (VRE) was once a simple pleomorphic organism that has now become extremely virulent because of antibiotic abuse. The pathogen of the 1990s is a bacterium that was harmless until transmutated by antibiotics. A clean kitchen sink keeps maggots at bay, not a coating of pesticide! If there is nothing rotten to attract flies they cannot lay eggs there. Yet part of our terrain is quite active and involves friendly life colloids like spores, bacteria, and yeasts that live in symbiotic relationship with us.

Healthy immunity has certain blood factors like acid/alkaline balance and blood inhibitors. Blood inhibitors are composed of organic substances like abascisic acid, tyrosinase, cyanhydric acid (Vitamin B17), diastastic poisons, and minerals like brass, lead, and mercury. These blood factors, as part of the immune system, keep blood young by inhibiting the evolution of the life colloid. They keep it to its first three allowable saphritic life forms and inhibit it from assembling into its more advanced pleomorphic stages, which may manifest as bacterium, bubble mycoplasma, yeast, ascospore, mycelial fibrous phallus, and others. Blood inhibitors keep life colloid evolution in the first three stages of its lifecycle, the healthy youthful stages that complement us. In these early three stages, the life colloids' later life forms such as mold, fungus, yeast, and acid-fast cell-wall deficient bacteria (cancer microbes) are inhibited by the body's dynamic vital terrain.

Healing a trauma to the body requires exudates (body fluids) and cells to pack into the area of injury and to create a fermentative process. Friendly forms of ferments (spores, double spores, and bacteria) produce substances that assist us, as well as other substances that are antagonistic to unfriendly forms. Friendly life forms help keep the body in an oxidative metabolism. The unfriendly forms are involved in fermentative decomposition of the body.

Colloidal nutrition in the form of friendly ferments produces beneficial dextrogyral (+) lactic acids. Friendly ferments produce helpful substances like glucuronic acid, usnic acid, B vitamins, free-form amino acids, and others. Unfriendly ferments produce detrimental levogyral

(-) lactic acid as a byproduct of their metabolism. Beneficial ferments and aerobic/anaerobic acidophilus help produce substances that bind to environmental and metabolic poisons, making them miscible with water and more easily swept out of the body. Immune cells of the body, friendly ferments, and microbes disassemble life colloids from unfriendly life forms within us, then either assemble them into oxidative healthy cells or direct them into the channels of elimination.

Friendly Colloids of Life Live within Us

There is a direct relationship to our health and the billions of beneficial microorganisms living in our intestines and on our skin. These friendly space dust critters provide a rich source of dynamic nutrients. They clean our colon of wastes and unfriendly critters, from harmful bacteria, to mold, fungus, and yeast, to other poisons.

You can receive help virtually overnight for seizures, diabetes, arthritis, pneumonia, Parkinson's disease, and immune challenges by simply ingesting soil-born organisms as a supplement. People have lived in such a sterile, antiseptic environment that these necessary symbiotic organisms have been missing in their diet. Most everyone can benefit from this supplement to seed the digestive tract from the mouth through to the rectum.

Primitive Life Eats Tar and Resin

Mineral colloids that make up asphalt eventually become life colloids (bacteria). These bacteria will ultimately digest the colloids that make up the rest of the road into space dust. Organisms considered to be foreign to our human system can provide genuine and dramatic health benefits from digestive, immune, and blood challenges through the ingestion of soil-born organisms.

Soil-born organisms, like phytoplankton and other microbes, have enzymes, hormones, and building blocks for vitamins (auxons), natural antibiotics (pacifarins), and many other nutrient byproducts. They also produce several intrinsic factors for the assimilation of vitamins and minerals. The microorganisms that colonize our lower intestine help us by transforming many nutrients into absorbable forms. People on a skeletonized cooked diet live with castings of hardened mucoid fecal matter adhering to their intestinal walls.

Living soil-born organisms—phytoplankton, acidophilus, and lichens—get in behind those laminated castings and crystallized acids and lift them off the intestinal wall, disassembling and dissolving all that mucoid matter. They turn the toxic mass of tar and resin-like substances into a bountiful harvest of enormous benefit in the form of a colloidal protein-derived biomass that our intestines can finally absorb. Assimilation and peristalsis is greatly enhanced as the intestines finally become clean and flexible after years of having to work on denatured foodstuff rather than fresh living LifeFood Nutrition.

Phytoplankton Turns On Immunity

Phytoplankton and other colloids of life found living on the outside of fresh fruits and vegetables assist our bodies with an enormous variety of tasks. Phytoplankton produces intrinsic factors that help with the absorption of nutrients and actually signal the stomach to produce hydrochloric acid necessary in digesting foods. These critters produce many proteins, some of which act as antigens that stimulate the amalwa cells. Amalwa cells are lymphoblastic cells of the thymus that are virtual cradles for the super fighting T and NK lymphocyte immune cells. When stimulated, they produce some twenty known species of alpha interferon, which supercharge the immune system.

Alpha interferon is a polypeptide for turning the whole immune system on! Each species of alpha interferon is produced for a specific antigen. The release of alpha interferon is so helpful as it produces and activates an enormous amount of granulocytes, leucocytes, phagocytes, and antibodies. Therapeutic doses of soil-born organisms have been shown to raise alpha interferon levels by 200 international units!

Life colloids as phytoplankton (space dust) are the substrate colloids for soil-born organisms and all other organisms. Phytoplankton become active after a long sleep if they are introduced into a solution of water or if they break free of more solid matter and become suspended in the air as dust. Friendly soil-born organisms introduced through LifeFood or supplements will cleanse the lower intestine and eat unfriendly opportunistic yeasts like candida albicans, along with all the other less than friendly organisms.

An antibody is created as an protein molecule (antigen) from either a phytoplankton or a soil-born organism, and then connects with either a white blood cell (leukocyte) or an amalwa immune cell. These cells are stimulated to produce an abundance of antibodies from this primal material. These antibodies are absolutely amazing because they can be stored in the body uncoded, until a time when they are needed by the immune system. When the immune system is challenged it simply draws upon this reservoir and imprints the uncoded antibodies with the precise information needed to transform the specific dysbiotic situation. By ingesting soil-born organism supplements, you can maintain an enormous reservoir of precious uncoded antibodies that stand ready to transform any pathogens you may come in contact with.

Untapped Antibodies and Metabolic Keys

Colloids of life produce intrinsic factors for the absorption of minerals and trace elements; for example, an iron-binding protein like lactoferrin is very important for iron absorption and storage. One should use this factor as a metaphor for absorption and storage of an enormous variety of nutrients. Iron-related metabolic health challenges can be solved by living the way nature intended—and occasionally eating a little dirt (soil-born organisms)—thus deriving benefits through this imprinting and through resonance. If iron from the diet is stored incorrectly it will cause corrosion. Corroded iron without proper levels of lactoferrin will also become available for unfriendly life colloids like candida albicans and other dysbiotic parasites. . Lactoferrin is the first corrective action taken by the body to properly store iron and keep its terrain intact.

Getting back to nature and eating some soil-born organisms encourages nerve growth and colony-stimulating factors to bring dramatic healing and extraordinary vitality. These dust critters provide us with a source of DNA and RNA from which we can produce almost everything else, from soil-born life colloids to all kinds of amino acids and other super nutrients. We even obtain all kinds of cellular benefits from their byproducts, such as the amazing antioxidant Super Oxide Dismutase (SOD).

SOD happens to be a byproduct of soil-born organisms, as is glutathione peroxidase. SOD and glutathione peroxidase help us to maintain excellent liver, blood, and lymph vitality, joint health and flexibility, ease of movement, immune function, and cardiovascular health. These byproducts also protect us from a variety of pathogenic situations involving the reduction of free radicals like cancer, arthritis, rheumatism, auto-immunity, hypertension, hepatitis, and other conditions. Soil-born organisms contain elements such as carotenes and bioflavanoids, along with pigments like chlorophyll. Space dust critters like phytoplankton provide us with the building blocks to make hormones, like Gamma Linolenic Acid (GLA). These critters even break down synthetic hydrocarbons—pesticides.

We are closest to the colloids known as enzymogens. Since we utilize elements in a manner where the life colloids are imbued with the vibration of having been part of a biological substratum, they can be stored and activated at any time. Typically, soil-born organisms require the naturally occurring minerals that functioned as co-factors where these plants once grew. These minerals include nitrogen, phosphate, calcium, magnesium, sulfur, boron, manganese, iron, copper, zinc, chloride salts, and molybdenum. Cultured soil-born organisms contain a variety of phytoplankton and lichens of the blue-green pigment families. These are minerals that can be taken as a whole food complex supplement.

Soil-Born Organisms Equal Food for Humans

Soil-born organisms produce proteins, carbohydrates, sugars, nitrogen, carbon dioxide, and other inert byproducts such as gases and water. Soil-born organisms and phytoplankton from LifeFood help to revitalize digestion, assimilation, and metabolism, and also invigorate the immune system with vital super nutrients. A commitment to LifeFood Nutrition, with a program of *electric* herbs (see herbal formulations, Chapter 11) and soil-born organisms for three to six months, can have the effect of clearing and restoring vision. Soil-born organisms give us the material for incredible flexibility, strength, and endurance. These friendly organisms snack on candida albicans and other unfriendly organisms, including penicillin and mucoralae (molds). Friendly organisms produce environments that pathogens cannot thrive in. This process is called bioecology (eco-sterilization). Rich nucleic acids, proteins, and pigments make friendly organisms extremely beneficial for health! Imagine reprogramming cells' metabolic mechanisms. Micronutrient presentation integrated into phytoplankton during its germination is like software for reprogramming the assimilation processes of mineral-starved cells.

Friendly life colloids coming from properly fermented and unpasteurized foods produce condensed, cationic colloidal minerals in the form of dextrogyral (+) lactic acid. They are life colloids at a primitive stage of their cycle. A few of these foods are kombucha, seed cheeses, L. Salivarius, unpasteurized sauerkraut, lemon cabbage elixir, *Rejuvelac*, raw apple cider vinegar, and soil-born organisms. Primitive life colloids bond with life colloids that comprise more advanced pleomorphic structures, like fungus, to disassemble them into more primitive life colloids. In that more primitive state, colloids lyse into a white snow or paste substance and then leave the body through all the channels of elimination, especially through the eyes, nose, ears, skin, tongue, vagina, and rectum.

Kombucha has life colloids of a friendly form called saccharomyces.

Saccharomyces reproduces by fission, unlike candida albicans that reproduces by spores. Friendly ferments and bacteria like saccharomyces cerevisiae and bifido bacterium (similar to acidophilus) are antagonistic to unfriendly ferments like ascomycetes of candida, mildew, penicillin, ergot, bread molds, e. coli, giardia lamblia, and entameba histolyticus. Giardia lamblia and entameba histolyticus live encysted outside the body for a couple of weeks, until consumed, at which point they pass right through the acid of the stomach to assemble into trophozoitic forms. Giardia migrates and colonizes in the small intestine and entameba in the colon. These are unsanitary illnesses and a good measure of hygiene goes a long way here. Giardia infections occur when domesticated animal feces leak into drinking water. L. Salivarius and soil-born organisms eco-sterilize. Everything has to be kept in balance. Even too much oxygen can bring on oxygen narcosis.

People eat foods contaminated with molds and fungi that, throughout their lifecycle, have released more than one thousand mycotoxins like acetaldehyde. Acetaldehyde condenses into acetic acid, lactic acid, uric acid, and ethyl alcohol. Those toxins disrupt blood colloidal homeostasis causing arteriosclerotic plaque, excessive low-density lipoproteins, or amino acid damage, conditions that cause poor blood and fluid colloidal integrity, blood vessels that are not intact, and an unhealthy pancreas, brain, and other organs.

Blood Protein and Colloidal Health

In live blood cell analysis, we prick the finger of a healthy hydrated person and the blood beads, standing tall as a little drop that indicates excellent blood protein colloidal homeostasis. Unhealthy blood contains colloidal challenges that are revealed when the ball of blood shows poor integrity and spills from the sides to smear on the slide. Acidic tissue and bloods that has lost its proper acid base sets the stage for fermentative conditions and germinative cancer cells (primitive fetal trophoblastic) to arise, compromising the immune system.

The challenge to restore vital health is found in protein and mineral digestion and assimilation. Poor choices of food cause major metabolic challenges; for instance, if a person eats cooked severely denatured food rather than LifeFood, we find coagulated, enzyme-resistant protein linkages that cannot mix with water (hydrophobic) because of a loss of enzymes, minerals, and vitamins.

Vital Pancreas Function Keeps Cancer at Bay

Pancreatic vitality can be formidably challenged without anionic colloids. Dead food is cationic and devoid of enzymes, thus robbing the body of metabolic enzymes needed for health. Chymotrypsin digests protein and is produced by the pancreas. Chymotrypsin is produced during sleep—the body's empty, restful, alkalizing stage—and naturally digests trophoblastic cells. Fluoride, which is added to half of the city water throughout America, compounds block Chymotrypsin formation!

Fetal trophoblastic (nutritional tissue) cells are a normal part of embryonic development. When sperm and egg meet, germinative trophoblasts are formed around it to nurse and protect the ovum. Simple life colloids from the father (spermatozoa) produce factors to protect the new growth of colloids from being disassembled by the mother's immune system. These spare life colloids assemble as trophoblasts, which then disperse and become incorporated into the embryo's colloidal structure.

Certain conditions like low oxygen or high estrogen levels, most especially the xeno-estrogens that modern pesticides are made with, cause colloids to assemble into trophoblastic forms. Cancer can be the result of pancreatic enzyme deficiency, estrogen present in a fermentative bodily terrain, or ecotopic (scattered) germinative trophoblastic cells. The liver ordinarily oxidizes estrogens, which is also supposed to be kept in balance by progesterone. When it goes wild this estrogen allows ecotopic-germinative-differentiated cells and undifferentiated simple fetal-trophoblastic cells to assemble into cancer.

The body usually has an array of strategies to handle trophoblastic cells—Vitamin B17 (amygdalin) for instance. Vitamin B17 is composed of glucose, benzaldehyde, and cyanide, and is found in more than a thousand fruits and vegetables. It keeps cancerous cells at bay, but it's also highly heat-unstable! Cancerous cells have an enzyme within them that releases both the benzaldehyde and the cyanide into the cell, causing its cache of colloids to be disassembled. Healthy cells lack this enzyme; plus they are surrounded by monatomic elements like rhodenase, which helps protect them from being disassembled (lysed) by this process.

Cancer Is a Single-Protein Disease

All disease results from a normal pattern of oxidative cell respiration becoming fermentative (anaerobic). Cancerous cells were cells that once existed without oxygen. They were cells that mutated back to their undifferentiated colloidal life form. Physical challenges, like consumption of heat-processed fats, proteins, and carbohydrates cause cells to lose their fixed voltage. This results in the occurrence of oxidation, fermentation, putrefaction, and rancidness in the body. The free radicals of disease lower the cells' electrical potentials.

Cancer occurs when the blood loses its proper acid buffers and becomes more alkaline than its usual pH of 7.3, exceeding 7.56. An excellent level of dextrogyral (+) lactic acid leads to proper oxidative cell respiration. Poor cell respiration and fermentation of blood sugar produces a buildup of a particular kind of lactic acid called a racemic mixture. That type of lactic acid is composed both of dextrogyral (+) and levogyral (-) lactic acids, which uniquely cancel each other out. That buildup promotes more fermentative development of the terrain.

Alkaline/acid balance influences each cell's morphogenic field, electrically influencing the cells to have greater or lesser voltages than those that would allow fermentative life colloids (trophoblasts) to exist. Cancerous cells arise because acid-fast cell-wall deficient bacteria help turn the terrain of the body and consequently its cells toward fermentative phosphorylation of ATP (energy).

As the electrical voltage of a cancerous cell's respiratory cycle is lowered or raised, it takes the it past its primitive stage back to its building block stage. It may also take the cell forward to its specialized stage, where the tertiary structure of its DNA shifts. Colloids of anaerobic cells, when they lose their voltage, disassemble (lyse) to become amino acids that are excreted out of the body in a snow-like catarrh. This discharge appears in urine and all other bodily excretions. If this voltage is raised, as in an alkaline body, colloids reassemble themselves into proper body cell architecture and function.

Sweating helps balance our pH through excreting L-lactic acid. Glucose fermentation is characteristic of cancer where the cells are starved for oxygen. Damaged DNA of cancer cells can be repaired with a reversal of fermentative, substrate-level phosphorylation toward oxidative energy (LifeFood), creating normal cell architecture and function.

Vitality Reveals an Alkaline Hyperoxia

Restoring vitality requires the presence of an alkaline hyperoxia, whereas disease involves acid hypoxia. Numerous biological factors are involved in the development of cancer, including the loss of dextrogyral lactic acid and an abnormal buildup in the tissue of levogyral lactic acid. Bringing dextrogyral lactic acid into the body and maneuvering other variable factors, like tissue pH and oxygenation, can favorably influence vitality.

LifeFood and an alkaline hyperoxia allow glucose to be metabolized to produce energy (ATP) with dextrogyral lactic acid as a byproduct. In the presence of oxygen, this lactic acid is converted into the more inert substance of pyruvic acid, which is used again in the storage of glucose as glycogen. In an acid hypoxia, however, glucose is fermented to produce energy (ATP) by becoming pyruvate and acetaldehyde. Fermentative life colloids have used acetaldehyde mycotoxins as a hydrogen acceptor and have made ethyl alcohol mycotoxins as a byproduct!

Cell energy production with dextrogyral (+) lactic acid ionizes harmoniously with anions to maximally create energy in the conversion of glycogen into energy and oxygen into mechanical energy. Glycogen is the principle carbohydrate stored in the body, even though levogyral (-) lactic acid mostly from cooked food creates less than vital, normal cell metabolism. Yeast, mold, and fungus are the principle undertakers, reducing all living things into the colloids of life that recycle, as all life does, and from which we are assembled. While someone has good vitality, the undertakers are kept at bay; otherwise we meet our fate: *from dust we come and to dust we shall return.*

Electric Nutrients Keep Our Terrain Intact

Eat fresh fruits and vegetables and unpasteurized ferments, like raw sauerkraut, to avoid damage from biochemical's and the mycotoxic wastes of yeasts and fungi, such as cyclosporin. In fresh fruits and vegetables, nuts, seeds, and friendly ferments you get antioxidants and whole-food vitamin/mineral complexes including:

- Vitamin A
- Vitamin C
- Vitamin E
- all B vitamins
- Vitamin K
- octocosonol
- Vitamin U
- methionine
- flavanoids
- soil borne organisms
- microhydrin
- selenium
- silica
- glutathione peroxidase
- superoxide dismutase
- cystine
- tocotrienols
- sulfur
- co-enzyme Q10
- lipoic acid
- bitter melon extract
- superzymes
- long- and short-chain essential fatty acids

THESE NUTRIENTS HELP BUILD our cells and our biochemical- and vibrational-mediated immune systems. They also help to alkalize and oxygenate the body. Cooked denatured food robs us of vitality and it leaves an acidic residue

155

The terrain of our bodies is maintained at 80 percent alkalinity and only 20 percent acidity. . The terrain of an apple is complete while its skin is intact; likewise, you are alkaline while your terrain is intact. Acute cleansing reactions are the body's attempts to mobilize mineral reserves in the healing process. Disruption to this ease in the body occurs when this alkaline balance is disrupted.

Body Chemicals Regulate Inflammation

Molecules of natural immunity are continuously being discovered. Some of these molecules represent chemokines excreted by the white blood cells involved in disassembling pathogens and neutralizing other immune challenges. Chemokines have also been of major importance in autoimmune inflammatory challenges like arthritis and lupus. Chemokines are the information molecules (proteins) that organize inflammatory cells.

Cells release chemokines to sequester materials needed to neutralize and disassemble antigens and pathogens. Selectins (proteins) lining blood vessel surfaces close to the infection bristle like burrs. White blood cells are drawn out of the blood seemingly by these selectins they stick to while they roll along the inflammatory vessel wall.

Chemokines drawn to blood vessel walls in the inflammation interact with white blood cells, making their surface membranes slightly abrasive with integrins. This altered surface provides the white blood cell with the traction needed to push through blood vessel walls. White blood cells follow a trail of chemokines through body tissue to the inflammation.

Chemokines signal white blood cells to excrete protein-derived enzymes to dissolve a path for the white blood cells to travel along. When the body is working well, with enough pH buffers and blood factors, immunity works well, with chemokines carefully orchestrating this immune response.

Macrophage proteins in lung inflammations are a factor involved in irreparable and formidable challenges of vital well being that can cause severe congestion. For that matter, any unbalanced situation, such as an imbalance of pH buffers, can encourage chemokine processes to become involved in disease.

Chemokines are one class of a number of information substances secreted by immune cells. Immune cells heal by excreting opiates and other peptides that make everything work. Science now understands that body function is a consequence of numerous information substances modulating brain function, like the polypeptide colloids (short-chain amino acids) assembled by gut, glial, immune, and nerve cells.

Physiological reactions take place as information substances connect with cell receptor sites throughout the body. This polypeptide system acts like a secondary nervous system. Immune cells excrete endorphins (happy information substances) and also have receptors for endorphins that modulate cell immune response. Minerals, hormones, alkaline body fluids, and a vital tissue pH of 6.8 are integral for DNA and RNA replication of many of these substances.

Cells and Biochemically Mediated Immunity

Cell-mediated immunity often overshadows another type of immunity called our biochemical defense system. Fragments of this latter system have been visible, yet with the recent discovery of anti-neoplastons, this system has taken more concrete form. Antineoplastons are medium to small peptide and protein derivatives that, through their harmonics, induce neoplastic cell colloids (cancer) to disassemble and reassemble themselves into vital cell architecture and healthy functional form. Healthy blood and urine has two types of antineoplastons, one with a broad spectrum of activity and one with a narrower spectrum of biochemical immunity.

Antineoplastons reprogram cancerous cells. Antineoplastons seem to act more with cells through information pathways, whereas most other immune components are purely energetic, involving larger molecules like antibodies. The major effect of cell-mediated immunity is through the energy of life colloids recognizing and neutralizing antigens, whereas antineoplastons reprogram cancerous cells through information substances. Protein colloids in urine have been in use in medicine since at least the first millennium B.C. There are an enormous number of pleomorphic growth inhibitors in urine. Even the medicine people of ancient America understood the application of urine in the treatment of cancer as it is used today.

Antineoplastons that are synthesized in the tissue are passed into the blood and urine. Much could be said about this biochemical immune system; one should be aware of the importance of such factors as acid/alkaline balance and colloidal health of the blood and of biochemical substances like glucuronic acid, abascisic acid, tyrosinase, and hydrogen peroxide that keep us healthy. All these elements are part of the biochemical immunity helping to keep our terrain intact.

Electric Foods Boost Immunity through Minerals and Hormones

Cultures living close to the Earth require at least fifteen types of vegetation per week to guarantee that they are getting the ninety minerals and various other phytochemical colloids needed to support excellent health. On one hand, you need mineral colloids plus hormones to mount an inflammation reaction necessary contain local lesions and manage early infections. Growth hormone from the pituitary, together with adrenal cortex mineral regulatory hormones (primarily aldosterone), acts as an alarm, signaling the immune system to contain noxious elements by initiating an inflammation. On the other hand, glucocorticoids are employed as anti-inflammatory hormones. A couple of the glucocorticoids are adrenal corticotrophic hormone of the pituitary and cortisol of the adrenals. The adrenals are involved in regulating metabolism of carbohydrates, fat, and protein. Seeds, nuts, roots, and bee pollen all have plant hormones and colloidal minerals that feed the pituitary and adrenals. Plant hormones make our immune colloidal mineral reserves mobile and usable.

Electric foods, which can grow in the wild, help alkalize the body, allowing for high amplitude of electricity. A few of these electric foods are: burdock root, apricot, dandelion greens, bee pollen, figs, kelp, dulse, almonds—and so many others. Throughout civilization, agriculture has taken wild plants and cross-bred them to make hybrids, enhancing their qualities for travel durability and shelf-life longevity, but sacrificing their biochemical means to survive in the wild, their vital electrics. For example, potatoes, grains, legumes, corn, carrots, beets, pineapples, kiwis, seedless grapes, and watermelons are all hybrids that lack vital electrics.

As long as the body has excellent vitality, its local defenses are sufficient. However, if the body is stressed by multiple infections and local defenses are less than adequate, the pituitary will release ACTH that stimulate the adrenals to flood the body with anti-inflammatory hormones.

In a compromised immune system, the ability to react with an inflammation response is low and lymphatic and thymus tissue shrink as the number of immune cells (lymphocytes) are reduced. This is an adaptive response, given a lack of resources that hinder enzymes from being able to completely help clear immune complexes. It indicates a fatty liver that is too compromised to correct the situation. Everything is fine as long as levels of enzymes and biological transmutation are adequate, which results from appropriate levels of hormones and minerals.

If immune complexes remain with enzymes after an inflammation rather than being disassembled by phagocytic life colloids (blood cells), they are deposited between the cells and activate an acidification of nitrogen that instigates a variety of symptoms. Bringing in hormonal and mineral colloids as they are needed is important in helping to restore the adrenal balance between inflammatory and anti-inflammatory hormones. This is where herbs and LifeFood are important and why other modalities are bound to have only limited success.

Body Cells Are Continuously Replaced

Liver cells are completely replaced every three weeks. Some cells, like endothelial cells, are replaced daily. Endothelial cells are the cells that line our passageways, including the mouth, nose, lungs, arteries, endometrium, and stomach. The least understood defense system in the body is the immune-lymphatic tissue of the reticulo-endothelial system (RES). Its component cells are dispersed throughout the organs of the body with single cells lining the lymph channels of the liver, thymus, lung, spleen, skin, bone marrow, adrenals, pituitary glands, and central nervous system.

Adaptive mechanisms of RES deal with stress by maintaining enzymatic, chemical, and hormonal balances in the body. Through white blood cells they orchestrate and maintain metabolism by immunologically healing and protecting. Good nutrition, like the fresh life colloids in LifeFood, is crucial in securing a tonified reticulo-endothelium and endothelial system (cells that line our passageways) whose cells need continual replacement. Again, an alkaline field is needed to build and protect these cells.

Unfriendly microorganisms replicate in body tissue with a fermentative acid pH. Friendly organisms exist in an oxidative and alkaline pH. Although the colon, bladder, mouth, and skin require a slightly acidic pH, most microorganisms can't thrive in an oxidative medium. Alkaline body fluid creates optimal energy as it emits a negative electromagnetic field.

Freedom from unfriendly microbes can be achieved through exposure to a relatively constant negative magnetic field for two weeks. Cancer can require up to twelve weeks of continuous exposure. This is what "electric" herbs and LifeFood nutrition do. This negative field produces greater amplitude of electricity, more alpha and theta states (slower and more organized electrical pulses), bicarbonates, and better liver and pancreas function.

Healing and maintaining vitality requires alkaline fluids and "electric" foods and herbs. Enzymes are life and they require electromagnetic energy for activation. Hydrogen peroxide is metabolized by catalase and colloidal metals, especially calcium and magnesium. An alkaline body allows essential minerals and amino acids to remain soluble and ionized. They are insoluble in an acid medium, where minerals will crystallize into insoluble complexes and amino acids will become a gel.

Electrons in an acid pH have been drawn from oxygen. In an acid medium, oxygen lacks any spare electrons and exists as peroxide. As long as that peroxide exists in an acid terrain, it cannot be reduced (given electrons) to oxygen and water. When the body is alkaline and oxygenated, vital immunity is at its peak. Some dysbiotic organisms within the body are oxidized (electrons drawn away from them), while others are reduced (given electrons) to neutralize them. The body in an alkaline state is fit to neutralize wastes from metabolism and dysbiotic organisms (mycotoxins). Acid waste is reduced only by alkaline body fluids.

Good vitality can be demonstrated to routinely involve conditions that keep minerals soluble. Electricity creates solubility. The more alkaline a solution is, the greater its amplitude of electricity. The moment electricity leaves a glass of juice, sediment forms on the bottom of the glass. Likewise, minerals in the body can become sediment, causing arthritis, arteriosclerosis, spinabifida, sclerosis, and rheumatics. These conditions are less of an overall calcium deficiency than a lack of calcium in the body where it *should* be and a congregation elsewhere where it *shouldn't* be.

Calcium needs to be in an anionic or cationic state in order to be used for specific metabolic tasks. These electrical forms of calcium benefit the body in unique ways. Many health practitioners have stressed supplementing with an iron that is cationic. What the individual with iron deficiency really requires is calcium in a special form and soil-born organisms. These would help in the absorption of required iron.

The Principal Undertakers
Are Mold, Fungus, and Yeast

Electric foods are the most important component of healing. They make the body alkaline. These are foods that grow in the wild. Today's huge hybrid carrot lacks vital electrics; it has to be nurtured in its growth. All commercially grown hybrid crops are missing their complete electrics. All these hybrid foods contain starch, a substance only found in hybrid foods. Fruit can be condensed into syrup, whereas starch condenses into paste.

Fruit syrup can be used to preserve, whereas yeast, mold, and fungus arise directly from starchy paste. The vitality of fruit is less available when eaten with starch because the mold, yeast, and fungus eat its simple sugars. Cells become swollen because of allergies to substances people consume, making the cells unable to absorb available nutrients. Those unused nutrients feed yeast, fungus, and mold to unfriendly microbes. These principle undertakers' primary function is to return all living beings to the space dust from which they come—us included. One can maintain excellent vitality by eating radiant LifeFood and leaving all hybrid food and starch out of the diet.

LifeFood and Electric Herbs Heal Cancer

New skin grows underneath an old mole or wart, causing them to dry and wither until they fall off. The same is true for all cancers in the presence of a beneficial negative electrical field. Cancerous cells are either dissolved by our blood or expelled. You can cleanse the body of acids in the tissue through LifeFood, "electric" herbs, and alkaline water, all of which create a negative magnetic field. Typically, people who successfully heal themselves heal their blood by bringing in specific blood-born inhibitors that block pleomorphic expression by allowing only oxidative phosphorylisation organisms and cell metabolism to exist.

We restore blood with electric herbs that alkalize body tissue and set up a negatively charged healing electrical field that constricts the passageways that feed cancers. This energy field is refreshing and oxygenating and provides for a biological reduction of all types of acid wastes, ranging from metabolism byproducts to mycotoxins, nu-toxins, and environmental toxins. Cells gradually revert back to their pristine order in the presence of a negative, reticular magnetic field.

CHAPTER 11

The Healing Powers
of LifeFood and Electric Herbs

Blood Purification
and Lymph Revitalization Formula

3 parts Red Clover
1 part Chaparral
1 part Oregon Grape
1 part Red Root
2 parts Blood Root
1 part Prickly Ash
2 parts Pau D'Arco
1 part Cat's Claw
½ part Poke Root
1 part Pipsissewa
2 parts Burdock Root
1 part Sarsaparilla
1 part Licorice
1 part Horehound
1 part Blue Flag
1 part Buckthorn
1 part Cascara Sagrada
1 part Kelp
¼ part Cordyceps
¼ part Ganoderma
2 parts Anise

BLEND HERBAL MIXTURE WELL and store in a dark cool container (the refrigerator is fine). Take 1 heaping teaspoon once or twice a day as a fresh compound in juice, or hot or room temperature alkaline-charged water. For chronic conditions, take for 4 to 6 months for a deep rejuvenation of the blood and lymph. This also serves as a tonic to boost any immune conditions by taking 1 heaping teaspoon once daily for 2 to 3 months. These are adult dosages; for children reduce according to body size. Pregnant and lactating mothers should consult a health care provider before taking any herbs.

Rotation Schedule for Herbs

WITH MOST HERBS, AND EVEN vitamin supplements, we recommend you take them on a rotation schedule of five days on with two days off, and three weeks on with one week off. Two days a week you should skip your formula, and after three weeks you should skip a week.

Compounding these 21 herbs increases their therapeutic effect. The individual action of each herb is altered and individual constituents are enhanced. This synergy enables these herbs to have their greatest effect. This formula purifies the blood and vitalizes the liver, spleen, kidneys, bowel, lymphatic system, and skin. The herbs are used over an extended period of time as the entire blood stream is gradually detoxified. This formula also helps with digestion, assimilation, and glandular secretions.

Potent alkaloids contained in this blood formula target retroviruses by inhibiting reverse transcriptase, the enzyme used to transcribe viral genetics into genetics of cells. This fresh compound brings *electrics* to support deep immune functions and the body's natural defense mechanisms; and to invigorate cellular biochemical electromagnetic immunity. This stimulates skin respiration, blood and lymph circulation, kidneys function, and peristaltic activity of the colon.

Acting as a blood and lymph restorative, this fresh herbal compound stimulates healing in metabolism by repairing catabolic tissue and waste responses. In most conditions of illness waste needs to be eliminated and the base of the blood built up. This compound promotes drainage and elimination and provides nutritional antioxidant, anti-tumor, and antiseptic hygienic activity.

Three Cancer Elimination and Body Detoxification Formulas

One

1	part	Virginia Snake Root
1	part	Echinacea Root
1	part	Thuja
1	part	Astragalus
1	part	Yellow Dock
1	part	Celandine
1	part	Mistletoe
1	part	Venus Fly Trap
2	parts	Turmeric
1	part	Periwinkle
1	part	Wild Indigo
¼	part	Cordyceps
¼	part	Ganoderma

Two

2	parts	St. John's Wort
1	part	Black Walnut Hull (green)
1	part	Violet, Blue
1	part	Heal-All
1	part	Irish Moss
1	part	Myrrh
1	part	Goldenrod
1	part	Schizandra
1	part	Blessed Thistle
3	parts	Fennel
1	part	Mandrake
1	part	Fenugreek

Three

1	part	Catalpa Blend (0.8 bark + 0.2 pod)
1	part	Mimosa Bark
1	part	Trumpet Creeper Root and flower
2	parts	Sweet Gum Blend (0.7 bark + 0.3 leaf)
2	parts	Angelica, Garden Root
1	part	Celandine
1	part	Dulse
1	part	Bitter Melon

GRIND AND MIX YOUR HERBAL formulas individually and store in a sealed container in a dark cool place (the refrigerator is okay).

Dosage

TAKE 1 TO 2 HEAPING TEASPOONS in juice or water as a fresh compound. Rotate the Formulas. Take one formula as a fresh compound for one week, resting from it two days a week. Then move to the next formula and take it for one week in the same way, rotating to the third. Rest the fourth week and then begin again with the first formula. Rotate through the formulas until the cancer condition is reversed. These formulas can also be used for general deep body detoxification by taking ½ to 1 teaspoon daily for several months.

Rotation Schedule for Herbs

AS STATED BEFORE, WITH MOST HERBS, and even vitamin supplements, we recommend you take them on a rotation schedule of five days on with two days off, then three weeks on and one week off. So, two days a week you should skip your formula, and after three weeks you should skip a week.

LifeFood Colloids and Cell Normalization

1) Phytochemicals neutralize the formation of carcinogens by completely blocking them and diverting them to a more stable metabolite.

2) Phytochemicals in LifeFood diffuse carcinogenic reactions with DNA by intercepting and helping metabolize carcinogens for transformation, metabolism, or excretion.

3) LifeFood colloids help in DNA restoration, such as in instances with amygdalin and Vitamin B17.

4) LifeFood colloids help give the body a chemical mediated immunity through antioxidant activity. They help with inflammatory and

anti-inflammatory activity through bringing spare electrons and reducing cancer-promoting agents.

5) The phytochemicals in LifeFood colloids keep toxicity away and out from the toxic compounds away from critical areas of the body. This happens in three basic ways:

    a) Phytochemicals chelate with toxic species and causes simple life colloids to become harmless. It neutralizes them.

    b) Phytochemicals activate the detoxifying enzyme systems.

    c) Phytochemicals from LifeFood inhibit catalytic reactions of toxic compounds.

Phytochemicals in LifeFood

Glucarates, curcumin, flavons, tannins, organosulfides, aromatic, isthicyanates, phenols, lignins, ellagicacid, saponins, esters, and ketones.

PHYTOCHEMICALS ARE plant-derived chemicals that help reduce oxygen free radicals. The active phenolic and polyphenolic compounds in various plants are potent antioxidants and activate detoxifying enzyme systems. Phytochemicals, like Omega-3 fatty acids in plants, also inhibit tumor formation by diverting damaging effects of arachidonic acid.

Some agents that are effective in blocking tumor promoters include the tannins, flavanoids, arachidonic acid metabolism inhibitors, organosulfides, and protease inhibitors. Phytochemicals from LifeFood keep in check the neoplastic cancer cell-producing processes, such as the protease inhibitors and turpins, and aromatic isothiocyanates and arachidonic acid cascade inhibitors. The important actions of phytochemicals neutralize and inactivate endogenous and exogenous carcinogens, raise cell voltage producing cell differentiation, and inhibit proliferation of neoplastic cells.

Phytochemicals can be used to heal specific conditions. Some strategies for restoring vitality with LifeFood are adaptogens, alteratives, gene repairing, altering hormonal receptor phytochemicals, enzyme therapy, and antioxidants.

LifeFood has all of its antioxidant properties which help spare the liver. Glutathione, an important antioxidant enzyme, is efficiently maintained in the liver when antioxidants come in the form of LifeFood. Strange compounds that enter the body that will become insoluble with water when combined with compounds to make them hydrostatic (cytochrome P450) at the cell level (Phase 1 level) and glutathione transferase (Phase 2) in the liver. The latter converts toxic substances into harmless, easily excreted compounds that exit in the bile or urine.

Adaptogens are substances that help us balance and regulate things. For instance, the adaptogen ginseng functions to raise low blood pressure in one person and lower high blood pressure in another. It works as a supreme *adaptor* for whatever is needed in the body that consumes it. Some adaptogens are ginseng, Vitamin C, royal jelly, suma, reishi mushroom, and Virginia snake root. These are nutrients or phytochemicals that help enhance all systems to create health equilibrium by improving the immune system and digestion and assimilation of nutrients and overall cell respiration.

Saponins, polysaccharides, and flavanoids give us a vital force from within and modify biological response times for healing reactions. Alteratives are phytochemicals that act like steam shovels in eliminating waste and causing the body's blood plasma to have good integrity. Gene repairing nutrients stimulate interlukens and interferons thus gene repairing occurs by inhibiting enzymes that promote cancer growth. Certain phytochemicals can compete for receptor sites of various hormonally effected cancers.

LifeFood Colloids Create Good Hygiene

LifeFood colloids cause the body to clear and clean debris. We have some seventy-five grams of protein in our blood plasma that the liver regulates. Albumin is released by the liver at a rate that is set according to the osmotic pressure of the blood. We have red blood cells, white blood cells, somatids, and three blood plasma molecules: fibrin, albumin, and globulin.

Albumin is the super protein transporter, transporting nutrients and body waste. Each gram of albumin contains about 3 million trillion molecules that transport nutrients and waste to purify and respire brain tissues and act as a rich cache of amino acids in protein synthesis. These LifeFood herbal formulas promote good hygiene, which reduces antibodies (globulins) and white blood cells and allows osmotic room for the stress-relieving super protein carrier albumin. A simple reduction of ten grams of antibodies allows more osmotic room for albumin. High levels of albumin in the blood indicate a robust immune system and good constitution.

Cordyceps

Mineral/hormone activation occurs because of certain energetic properties in LifeFood colloids like those of the miracle mushroom, cordyceps. Cordyceps is a dry complex composed of the sclerotium of a fungus and the corpses of moth larvae. The fungus is parasitic to the larvae, which makes it an extremely unique food, indeed. It is used as a homeostatic, a mycolytic, and a diaphoretic and in respiratory conditions, as an expectorant and an anti-asthmatic. The life colloids in cordyceps are imbued with an intelligence that goes between minerals, phytoplankton, bacteria, mold, fungus, yeast, plants, and simpler and larger life colloidal organisms.

The cultured mycelia of cordyceps can boost a sluggish immune systems and make the immune and metabolic systems bristle with energy. This increases the size and integrity of the spleen and helps to heal an exhausted liver. Elements in cordyceps (cordycepin GP) increase the absorption of vital mineral colloids into endocrine glands and other vital organs. Cordyceps is also an excellent bronchial dilator because it increases airflow through the passageways of the lungs.

Electric Herbs Help Clear Cell Waste

Colloids come together to form a variety of nutrients from herbal formulas and work to assist the body's immunity by accelerating the white blood cells' response in disassembling unfriendly life colloids. The herbs help with the digestion of unfriendly life colloids by softening their membranes so that immune complements can stick to them. Immune cells produce complement proteins that stick to unfriendly life colloid membranes so antibodies can anchor themselves to the debris in need of disassembly. Some of the herbs speed up lymphocyte replication. The herbs help the body with peripheral circulation and to clear the trash floating around in health challenged tissue, thereby improving overall immunity and resolution.

Body tissue is made up of two basic types of cells: mesenchymal and parenchymal. Mesenchymal cells form vessels, glues, and structures. Even in a relatively polluted environment, they work to aggressively repair. They are durable and metabolically slower than parenchymal cells, which are involved in secreting, digesting, communicating, and contracting. Parenchymal cells have a higher rate of metabolism. They are more delicate and easily challenged to repair and reproduce when they're in a less than healthy environment.

Cells first begin healing with a change in body fluids as they become clean. Cells live within a packing material (mucopolysaccharide hydrogel) that acts like a hermecticant, drawing and holding water into itself. This process is a good arrangement because cells combust oxygen and glucose into water and carbon dioxide. Solid trash is drawn out of the cells away to lymphatic drainage. Blood platelets (fibrin, globulin, albumin) normally remain in the blood vessels. If they escape, they cause extended inflammation. If troublemaking dysbiotic life colloids dissolve the mucopolysaccharides, then cells expand and waste products back up and collect rather than being completely eliminated.

The polysaccharides in the herbal formulas assist to maintain the structure of water inside cells and also high nutrient integrity in the packing material contained within the body cells. These polysaccharides help hold the hydrogel together, preventing it from being dissolved. This aids immensely in the tissues' ability to heal because keeping water and waste streaming out of the cells makes space for needed chemical nutrients to be drawn in to run the machinery of the cell.

The electrical charge of our components allows the orderly flow of liquids (electrons) between exiting and entering blood capillaries. Nutrients are actively drawn in and waste products are passively swept and electrically drawn away from blood vessels toward lymph capillaries. Electrical elements in the herbal formulas encourage lymph drainage. Cellular colloidal waste is reassembled into usable colloids for storage and unusable colloids to be excreted.

The alkaline colloids of various herbs stimulate the quality of cellular membranes, repelling them from each other. A cell near the wall of a blood vessel, as with all blood plasma molecules, keeps to the center of the capillary. This arrangement allows for excellent exchange of nutrients and discarding of waste materials at the cell membrane surface. This surface interchange is between the cell's inside surface, facing toward the blood, and the outside surface of endothelial cells. The interchange is via interstitial fluids that flow into blood capillaries. In this arrangement the blood feeds the lymph. The lymph, in turn, nourishes body cells. Alkaline colloids in the herbal formula enhance the nutrients in blood to flow through lymphatic membranes. Having a negative redox potential in blood stimulates an eternal fountainhead of electrons, creating a nice flow and exchange of electrons. The electric herbs in the blood purification and cancer formulas are effective in disassembling unfriendly life colloids like mold, fungus, yeast, bacteria, and spores.

Bio-Resonance: Like Cures Like

Formulations, such as the Blood and Lymph formula, intensify innate body healing energy. Even elements in the formula like diastastic and cyanhydric poisons are vitalized nutrients when taken as a fresh compound. Vitalized energetic properties of LifeFood colloids activate their less energetic properties. Energy is transferred, through resonance, when similar vibrations are harmonically energized by the higher vibrations of vital life colloids.

Even the heavy metals and radioactive materials in LifeFood colloids are important. The higher vibrations of the heavy metals and radioactive elements in Celtic sea salt and Icelandic kelp provide essential harmonic bio-resonance that assists the body to clear away heavy metals of a lower order and vibration. Electrons spinning with bio-resonant deviance, like those in elements such as mercury, lead, uranium, and aluminum, are enlivened when in their natural vitalized state. All nutrients should come with their vitamin and mineral complexes intact, the way nature intended. Denatured food causes dysbiosis.

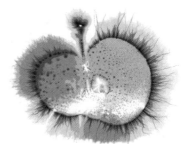

CHAPTER 12

Common Challenges

Candidia Dysbiosis

Today many people suffer from candida, a condition where a proliferation of yeast feeds on refined sugar in the blood and the sugar from starches in the body. This situation arises when there is an utter lack of friendly bacteria to keep yeasts in check and a lack of friendly ferments, like sauerkraut, in the diet. Many factors lead to these symptoms, the most major of which include loss of friendly bacteria through antibiotic abuse, flying in airplanes at high altitudes (bacteria are very temperature and altitude sensitive), long periods of extreme stress or emotional distress, a diet comprised of starches and sugar foodstuffs with a devastating lack of enzymes, and as stated above, a lack of friendly ferments in the diet.

Candida albicans is an unfriendly yeast that thrives in an oxygen-starved environment; oxygen is needed to help reduce acids. That situation requires proper respiration and revitalizing the adrenal glands and the mineral/hormone action mechanism. The medulla (our primitive or reptilian brain) increases sodium distribution, which in turn elevates blood sugar levels, adding to the plasma and cell starvation of oxygen. This usually causes dry mouth, general thirst, and salt cravings.

Alkaline hydration is important and the glucopoly-saccharides in LifeFood colloids, along with silica, help with this. Fresh urine, soil-born organisms, L. Salivarius, enzymes, and other LifeFood colloids may be necessary to help restore the body's vital terrain.

Animal-like fungal rods of candida contribute to the production of errant substances that produce an array of mental and physical challenges. These substances are aptly named exorphins and mycotoxins, respectively. Candida is a huge red flag for *needing a boosted immune system*. Life colloids as ferments are unique in larger organisms as well. Hippopotami and eagles both breathe air. Nevertheless, they are very distinct. The varieties of ferments are just as distinct as those of vertebrates. We find that yeasts derive their nutrients via enzymes, acting similarly to the roots of plants in the way they draw in nutrients. In a proper environment, one single yeast cell can become a hundred in one day. Candida has two recognizable forms—a yeast form and a fungal form. In its fungal form it assembles colloids into rhizoids (long root-like structures), which penetrate the tissue mucosa and bridge the boundary between the internal body and digestive tract. This is a very serious condition as the fungal/animal-like candida can create a tunnel out of the digestive tract (mouth to rectum) that can stream digestive material from the inside of the digestive tract to the interior cavity of the body. This horrible condition is the result of eating poorly, allowing all kinds of debris to constantly circulate in the bloodstream.

Immunity built of friendly life colloids and biochemical elements keeps those less than friendly colloids (like candida) at bay. Candida ferments sugar, reducing it to acetaldehyde! Sound LifeFood Nutrition that keeps candida out of the diet is required for maintaining vital immune function. Vital immunity needs minerals and hormones to be able to reassemble the yeast life colloids into healthy cell architecture and function. However, some individuals eventually become tolerant of unfriendly life colloids, indicating a situation of very low and compromised immunity.

You Have Electricity While You Are Alkaline

While we sleep, our electricity pulses between 0.5 and 2.5 times per second. During this time, our body switches to an alkaline phase. The central nervous system is electromagnetically negative, producing a south-seeking magnetic field. Our electrons spin in a counterclockwise direction. This stimulates the production of anabolic hormones, melatonin, and growth hormone. Catabolic hormone production is reduced to a low level during this phase.

As we sleep, we create an alkaline field in our bodies in order to grow, repair, and reduce acids. As we awaken, our electricity's amplitude decreases when its frequency goes above 12 cycles per second. Consciousness emerges around 22 cycles per second with fairly low amplitude. The more alkaline the body is, the greater the amplitude of electricity it has; the more acidic, the lower the amplitude of electricity. Alkalinity has a counterclockwise spin on electrons, whereas acidity has them spinning clockwise.

Alkaline electromagnetic fields encourage maximum phosphorylisation of ATP by oxidation and inhibit fermentative phosphorylisation. Alkaline blood allows for more complete protein synthesis. Anything that would allow a less oxidative medium in the body would cause a less than excellent level of protein synthesis. Alkaline tissues and blood convert acids and free radicals to water and oxygen. They create an antibiotic blood interface with dysbiotic pleomorphic organisms. Alkaline blood and tissues neutralize toxins, restoring and maintaining vitality.

Energy is released when anions and cations merge! Anions migrate toward the sunlight and cations toward the center of the earth. Excellent health requires an abundance of anionic food. The modern diet of cationic, denatured, skeletonized food has had quite the opposite effect. There are many anionic and cationic forms of calcium. Anionic calcium is found in vibrant leafy greens, while cationic calcium is found in pasteurized milk and the ground oyster shell calcium used for poor-quality mineral supplements.

Each colloidal mineral performs an important bodily function. Typically, fruits and vegetables growing toward the sunlight have anionic forms of calcium, potassium, and chlorine. Lemons are anionic because they have an abundance of alkaline elements, including calcium, sodium, potassium, and magnesium. Organs below the stomach require anionic energy to work, while the stomach itself requires more cationic energy (acidity) for optimal efficiency.

Acid/Alkaline Colloidal Interaction

Having an alkaline body dissolves solidified (acidic) calcium. When the body encounters an acid, a mycotoxin, or a nu-toxin, it uses calcium and other alkaline buffers to neutralize these acids. In an acid medium, that calcium becomes solidified, while in the presence of body tissue pH of 6.8 and blood pH of 7.3 that same calcium naturally dissolves.

Liquids that conduct electricity contain sodium and potassium. The outer electrons of potassium and sodium flow freely, allowing for a greater conductivity of electricity. Colloidal interaction affects your ideal weight and whether you have the tendency to gain or lose minerals. We should have the correct potassium to sodium relationship. This means we should have more potassium than sodium; more magnesium and silica than calcium; more iron than manganese; more copper than iron, and more zinc than copper. Potassium is often what we need more of. When the body has enough potassium inside every cell, the cell tissues allow the blood vessels to finally relax. The heart can then rest more easily. Magnesium helps with spare potassium. Vitamin B6 (in a whole-food vitamin complex) is very important. If extracellular fluids contain balanced sodium, then potassium stays inside the cells. Otherwise, the terrain becomes sullied. These fundamentals of the acid/base relationship are essential for healing.

Influencing the Absorption of Minerals

For minerals to be absorbable by the body they have to be in a colloidal form. They also need to have been part of a biological system, like algae, friendly bacteria, to be within their whole-food mineral complex such as you would generally find it in nature. Friendly bacteria biologically transmutate the mineral kingdom for us into colloids of a highly absorbable form. Colloidal minerals compete for absorption sites and carrier molecules. Calcium from mineral rock supplements, or from hybrid foods like carrots, are forms of calcium that have a totally different electron spin than the organic living calcium found in red clover blossoms.

Iron from a natural food like burdock root will spoil if mixed with iron from a carrot. This subtle though significant reaction occurs because the minerals compete for anionic ligands. Mineral colloids are also susceptible to being restricted by phytic acid from seeds and grain cereals. That joining renders them unavailable for intestinal absorption.

For absorption, the mineral colloid has to remain in its ionic state! Zinc and calcium are seriously challenged by the phytic acid content in the poor diet containing cooked, denatured, and skeletonized grains and legumes.

Chemically similar ions compete for the same transport carriers. Low molecular weight carrier proteins bind to the mineral to be transported. Everything has to be bound to a protein carrier to become miscible in body fluids. This interaction is excellent when electromotive potential can be engaged by its protein carrier. Colloidal minerals coming from a biological system, such as calcium kale or spinach, are imbued with a living active energy that mineral calcium from dolomite will never have because it is inorganic and inert.

Being Alkaline and Staying Trim

Fat dissolves in an alkaline medium. Most diets, however, are not even close to alkaline—they are in fact quite acidic! Free radicals and peroxides produce an inflammatory condition and acidic pH. Acids are stored in fat cells to keep the blood pristine. Needed weight loss only occurs when the body is brought into an alkaline medium. Alkaline nutrients from electric herbs and LifeFood Nutrition buffer inflammation and restore the body to its proper pH, creating the right environment for the reduction of fat and acid weight. Addictive withdrawal reactions are nothing more than various acids needing to be neutralized by oxidation (alkalinity and oxygen).

Amino acids and fatty acids come in two types: levogyral and dextrogyral. Levogyral amino acids and fatty acids (rotate plane polarized light to the left) are biologically compatible and support health (alkalinity), while dextrogyral amino acids and fatty acids are toxic (acidic) to the human body. Levogyral amino acids and essential fatty acids rotate polarized light in the same direction as the negative magnetic field of an alkaline body. It's interesting to note that left polarizing proteins and fats work toward oxidation and alkalinity, whereas right polarizing lactic acid (dextrogyral (+)) is involved in the conversion of sugar into glycogen (sugar stored in the muscles and liver) in the presence of oxygen.

Having an alkaline medium enhances greater amplitude of electricity in the body! Levogyral (-) lactic acid from cooked carbohydrates and denatured foods is involved in the fermentation to get energy. Cooked carbohydrates like bread and pasta causes a weaker field in the substrate, leaving levogyral lactic acid (-). That field is too low to match the anion spins of oxidative body fluid (pH 7.3–7.4) that is needed to support the energy required to achieve oxidation.

Alkaline-Hyperoxia versus Acid-Hypoxia

Alkaline-hyperoxia is required for neutralizing toxins and dysbiotic pleomorphic organisms, healing and repair, production of oxidation-remnant magnetization, and oxidative phosphorylation producing ATP (energy). Two sources of life energy are produced from oxidation—ATP and oxidation-remnant magnetism. Live biological cells produce ATP (energy substance). Crystals of magnetite are stored in the pineal gland, ethmoid magnetic organ, and in neurons. These crystals are made in cells by oxidative-remnant magnetism.

Immune challenges, enzyme inhibition, injurious addictions, toxins, and cancer are all symptoms that involve local acid-hypoxia. There is an alkaline-hyperoxia replacement of acid-hypoxia in the correction of acute symptoms, such as dissolving tumors and cysts. The restoration of vitality and the reversal of degenerative disease require an alkaline-hyperoxia. Cellular and tissue alkaline-hyperoxia is produced by the beneficial negative magnetic field from anionic colloidal nutrition.

Anionic colloidal nutrition, which produces a negative magnetic field, supports the bicarbonate buffer system involved in the direct maintenance of body alkalinity. Releasing oxygen from hydrogen peroxide and acids (oxy-acids) creates oxidative active molecular oxygen. This is made possible by either a negative magnetic field or an enzyme catalyst (oxidoreductase) as the energy activator. The blood requires proper colloidal integrity. Anionic mineral colloids are very important in this process. Excellent sources come from sea vegetables.

Life and the Balance of Mineral Colloids

Both a young and old bull whales have exactly the same ratio of minerals in their blood and plasma. All species of life, except for humans, have similar balanced mineral profiles between young and old. In humans, however, there is an enormous disparity when comparing the mineral profiles of a vital person and a person who has low vitality. Factors such as anionic or cationic, chelated organic and inorganic forms change the way minerals are absorbed. If minerals from wild foods—like iron from burdock root—were mixed with iron from a hybridized food like carrot, it would spoil the good iron's chance of absorption. Because the intestinal wall has a negative charge, it keeps positively charged minerals attracted to it. Therefore, it blocks passage of positively charged minerals into the bloodstream. Mineral colloids from sea vegetables and other forms of LifeFood Nutrition are naturally chelated with amino acids that shield their positive charges, allowing them to pass through the intestinal wall.

Small departures from the body's normal alkaline colloidal mineral composition can have consequences of profound physiological significance. Yet those changes may hardly make any appreciable difference to the whole body composition. The characteristic concentration and form should be maintained within narrow limits. If structural and functional integrity of tissues is safeguarded, then health, growth, reproduction, and repair functions remain vital. Mineral colloids are involved in enzymes activation (intracellular and extracellular), regulation of the pH levels controlling metabolic reactions, and cell osmotic homeostasis, all of which maintain the body's vital terrain.

Colloidal mineral and pH buffers, which the body only has in trace amounts, determine the person's overall vitality. For instance, zinc plays a vital role in protein synthesis, even though the concentration of zinc in the body is very small, only about 0.002%. Niacin is involved in placing zinc in DNA polymerase enzymes. Niacin, in conjunction with zinc, makes protein synthesis possible! Protein synthesis requires electrons, and other nutrients as well. The body is going to have plenty of spare electrons with a LifeFood life style. The LifeFood body easily maintains its alkalinity and negatively charged (-) electromagnetic field.

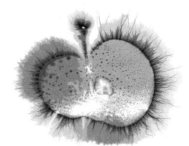

CHAPTER 13

The Cosmic Human

Light Opens Our Third Eye

The pineal gland is located deep in the brain and is responsible for, among other things, setting our sleep/activity cycles through secretion of melatonin. How much is secreted is influenced by how much rest and darkness a body receives. Melatonin helps the body move into an alkaline state when we go to sleep. While we sleep, anabolic steroids are released to help build up the body. Slowed breathing alkalizes the body. We have had a greater reliance breathing through the tubercles of the nose since the last pole shift 13,000 years ago. This, along with the measurable decrease in the Earth's magnetism over the last 200 years and a fresh awareness of kundalini yoga and pranic breathing, has brought attention to strange and interesting nutrients for the pineal gland—namely electrons, light, and photons.

The pineal gland's fuel source comes in primarily through the nose in the form of negative ions. Influencing this supraluminal energy, as it is harnessed from the ethos, is accomplished by breathing energy in through the soft part of the top of the skull, drawing it up through the feet and into the joints through the breath. Bringing blood to the farthest reaches by abdominal breathing oxygenates and alkalizes the body. This creates a feeling of pleasure that stimulates synchronization between the brain hemispheres and creates entrainment where a multitude of neurons act as one. Pleasure creates states of whole brain functioning. Whole brain functioning naturally alkalizes the body.

Our thoughts and feelings are continuously coding our nervous system. Moment by moment, our thoughts regulate our emotions and our physiological processes. Pleasurable thoughts stimulate the production of endogenous opiates to be released from where they are produced in the fourth ventricle of the brain. These endogenous opiates act like information substances; like a secondary nervous system regulating such diverse actions as turning the immune system on and off. This immune-modulating system is regulated through the breath and our breathing habits. Our "in the moment" thoughts are continuously modulating the whole immune system. For example, we often inhale powerfully and fill the entire lung when we feel pride or relish a victory, while the sad or depressed person may only engage his shallow breathing, causing him to be collapsed in the lung and ribcage, shoulders hunched forward.

All the systems of the body are affected by internal and external forces of nature. Cell nuclei swell and shrink at specific times during a twenty-four-hour period. There are personal, cyclical, and seasonal variations of energetic influences on our biological rhythms. Rhythms of the day are called circadian rhythms and are composed of two distinct types: endogenous and exogenous. The blood carries the forces of the ego. A person wanting to eat something sweet at a certain time produces endogenous opiates. Sweetness can allow the amino acid tryptophan to cross the blood/brain barrier, stimulating serotonin and melatonin to be produced. Even the level of serotonin, secreted by the pineal gland, has a twenty-four-hour cycle.

Ordinarily, we draw energy in from telluric and astral forces. Adaptations in our body that evolved over millions of years have shaped consciousness. Significant changes in the brain have occurred; for example, the pineal gland has been drawn into the deepest part of our skull, reflecting a time during our evolution when we were living through a semi-nocturnal phase. During times of geophysical planetary stress conditions, our organ functions change a bit as a result of conscious adaptation. The pineal gland, the size of a quarter 13,000 years ago, is now the size of a pea, becoming smaller as it becomes more sensitive.

The pineal gland is like a primitive eye, referred to as the "third eye" throughout history. The gecko has a pineal gland so close to the surface that is only sheathed by a layer of its skin. With its sensitivity to photons, it modulates the conductivity of light. This gland is fed with the energy it requires from our supraluminal plasma bodies. These bodies are influenced by thought as well as by geophysical conditions. The strength of the Earth's magnetic field has dropped from 4.0 to 0.5 gauss in the last 200 years, making it only 12 percent of what it was 200 years ago.

The ethmoid organ is involved in picking up micropulsations coming through the Earth's crust. Just like ringing a bell, there is an incredible resonance and vibration occurring on the Earth around physical matter that interacts with the ethos. The vibration of this interaction of matter with ethos is like a colloid suspended in the electro-supraluminal solution of the universe; it is both heard and seen. We draw energy from all around the body into the joints and the marrow of the bones. To consciously slow the breath down, we can affect the subtle energy around us with a simple focus on the inspirative aspect of breath coming in. This will calm the mind and emotions and enhance our absorption of the energetic matter of the universe.

Celestial Bodies Affect Minerals in Solution

The faster a planet is moving and spinning the more its corresponding metal is able to conduct electricity. Even inorganic colloids undergo periodic physical variations and change their properties over a few years or even in a single day. The official universally accepted weight for a kilo—a beaker composed of inorganic colloids—is under lock and key in a chateau outside of Paris. Only three people have a key to this room and twice a year they go and check the weight. It has baffled them to find that this beaker is gradually losing weight at the rate of the equivalent of a grain of salt each year. This beaker, however, is very much a part of this living, expanding and contracting, assymbling and disassymbling universe of moving colloids. Because the Parisians are firmly rooted in their belief that solid matter never moves they can't imagine what is happening. March and September happen to be the months these colloids are most affected because of the equinoxes. The earth is exposed to certain radiation belts due to the unique movement of our solar system. Celestial radiation affects biological systems considerably. Sunshine, sunspots, solstices and equinoxes, solar and lunar eclipses, and the daily and monthly cycles of the moon affect the tides of ions in the atmosphere.

Colloids are extremely sensitive to these celestial movements. The blood protein albumen changes its precipitation of flocculent when the Earth moves into line with a group of sunspots. When the moon eclipses the sun, flocculation is reduced. Fifteen minutes prior to sunrise there is an increase in flocculation that wakes the well rested and draws them into the day. This anticipation demonstrates hoe the body effectively acts as a sundial.

Energy Comes from Sources Other than Food

Minerals, hormones and other phytochemicals in plants are charged by the Earth's magnetic field. It's estimated that 70 percent of life energy comes from digested food. Energy is required to digest and assimilate nutrients. Under normal circumstances, it's estimated that the body uses about 30 percent of its energy expenditure for this purpose. Cooked denatured food would have cost the body greater energy in the long run—greater than 30 percent.

Exogenous energy sources are accounted for by the body's own magnetic field, in addition to direct sources like sound, light, and cosmic and telluric forces. Chemical remnant magnetism through oxidation produces magnetized crystals from iron and manganese. These crystals are the body's own lodestones that act to orient us with the north or south poles of Earth and give us a sense of direction. They can be found in the ethmoid organ, pineal gland, and in various nerve cells.

Even highly alkaline-charged water is pure and simple energy! Alkaline water dissolves acids.

Nutrients Have Strange and Interesting Qualities

Emotions run every physiological system in the body. Sweetness in disposition overstimulates (alkaline) pancreas function, whereas bitterness (acidic) can overstimulate stomach secretions. Currently, there is a vast void where mind meets matter in medicine, which thankfully is being filled by alternative healing therapeutics and preventative medicine. If one is happy, the brain and immune cells secrete happy information substances like endogenous opiates that go about boosting the immune system wherever it is needed. The subtle energies of our emotions change the energies of our overall physiology. Emotions trigger the simultaneous secretion of information substances all over the body! This is a very real effect that occurs directly through consciousness. When we feel rapture and great love the veins and arteries relax, dilate, and move blood; circulation is improved and the cheeks gain color. This opposed to when we feel judged, depressed, or ashamed, where blood flow slows, the breathing becomes shallow, and the face pales as veins and arteries constrict.

Light Is a Nutrient

Photons from the sun energize electrons in our body through resonance. Our body's colloids of light, which are the same size as a wavelength of visible light, are energized by supraluminal energies streaming out of the sun. This affects our plasma bodies instantly, even though light particles take eight minutes to arrive from their long journey from the sun.

Sunlight is an important nutrition. We eat half the food we normally would when we take in electron-rich elements. The pineal gland is exactly like an eye that has migrated into the darkest part of the head and like an eye is hollow with a lens that responds to brightness and color. The pineal gland regulates all inner light activities. Most all of, this light enters the body through the eyes and heads directly to the pineal gland for mediation.

Breathing and States of Consciousness

Opiates, polypeptides, and proteins are information substances that help tune and modulate the whole body. These information molecules are generated and influenced through breathing. One can change consciousness by hyperventilating or hypoventilating. Having more or less oxygen and carbon dioxide changes our body pH balance. Consciousness manifests itself through our breathing.

Inspiration is the act of inhaling air through the nostrils. Ideas come to us on the inspiration. In any blissful, joyous moment one can observe that there is more conscious attunement to the inspirative aspect of breath. Desirable hemisphere synchronization occurs as the heartbeat and the breath come into rhythm; you can tap into a literal sipping of abundant universal energy where electrons are being materialized all around us. If one has enough electrons one can appear immortal. It is electrons that animate us.

Pranic breathing harnesses our supraluminal energy. This energy is like a field in our plasma body with an energetic point of two types of energy coming together. This energy exists even inside a vacuum. It comes into the body one hand's width above the crown of the head and one foot's depth below the feet. Without water a person can live about six days; without food, for weeks. A person can live without oxygen for a few minutes; yet, the instant we disconnected with this supraluminal field, we die.

Astral energy enters through the soft plate at the top of the skull. Telluric forces join with our plasma body from below and come in through our feet. We have an electrical storm within and around us, with bolts of lightning that crackle all around. Our breathing, thoughts, and states of consciousness are major forces that shape our bioenergetic field.

Homeopathy is one type of medicine that is based on the fact that polypeptides are acted upon by subtle vibrational energies. Emotions run throughout the body. There is wisdom and interconnectedness in every cell. Many of the information substances, like neuropeptides, are found throughout the body and can also be found in the fourth ventricle, which is integral to where the control of breathing occurs. Released peptides regulate breathing, which in turn regulates our state of consciousness. One can change one's will in order to start a cascade of polypeptides that affects the emotional state, and also such diverse systems as the blocking of binding sites and virus spore growth.

Minerals do many amazing things for us. Iron allows us to love; sodium allows us to be flexible; silicon allows us to be elastic. Under the influence of the sun, plant chlorophyll can provide electrons to a semi-conductor such as zinc oxide. Even the life of chlorophyll can be extended by adding an electrolyte (hydroquinone) to its saline solution. Chlorophyll can act as an electron-producing pump to produce a kilo-watt of power from hydroquinone! Minerals help conduct electricity.

Water, which would ordinarily remain inside a capillary tube, begins to flow when the capillary tube is electrified. Nutrients like Co-enzyme Q10 give the body the ability to transfer electrons from one molecule to another. Electricity can affect the growth rate of colloids of life, and their subsequent structures as larger organisms, by altering the viscos-ity—the flow resistance—of fluids.

Magnetism draws oxygen and other nutrients into the blood and also into the most distant, deepest places inside the body. The integration of moisture is electronic. We grow from an abundance of electrons into the form of ourselves from water expressing itself. After all, we are mostly made of water.

Vitality can be likened to a matter of cells in oscillating equilibrium. Good health is seen when the vibrational strength or quality given off by healthy cells and life colloids is finer than the oscillation or vibra-tion of those less than friendly life colloids. A few minutes' exposure to the fingertips of a person with high-voltage, alkaline, electro-gravitic energy can disassemble unfriendly colloids like yeast even at a distance.

Primitive life forms converse with each other through electromagnetic rays. All colloids of life (and their larger organisms) become imbued by their ability to amplify and resonate with universal energy. This results in fields of fine subatomic sheaths which permeate the body.

Trace elements, like lithium—one of the lightest minerals known—help nerve action potential. Lithium can substitute for sodium in these action potentials. A person can have excess sodium chloride in the tissue and be thoroughly depleted of it in the blood at the same time. That condition comes from a diet of denatured, poisonous, heat-processed sodium chloride. Lithium is an element often found in nature around alkaline hot springs. It is very helpful in stabilizing moods. Lithium supports high-voltage slow-wave electroencephalic brain waves, superimposed with beta waves. Phytochemicals, phytoplankton, and their constituent cache of life colloids that come from plants, soil and algae are the raw materials that allow us to maintain our invisible reticular magnetic field.

The south-seeking end of the magnet (N-) pulls toward the center of a tornado and causes blood cells to spin in a counterclockwise direction, decreasing hydrogen ions and making us sweeter. That pole of the magnet that seeks north is the south positive end (S+), which pushes outward from the center and causes cells to spin in a clockwise direction, making us acidic and bitter.

Nutrients that are like the south-seeking end of the magnet (N-) are sweet and tend to slow things down (parasympathetic), while the north-seeking magnet pole, which is the south positive (S+) end, speeds things up (sympathetic). The ionic properties of nutrients relate to how well the body handles the hydrogen ion (pH). Nutrients help restore our magnetic field and restore and maintain other things in the body like maintaining the original pigment of hair.

Alkaline fluids with negative electromagnetic fields facilitate the body's ability to reduce acids and create ease in the transformation to total vitality. Cleansing reactions and addictive withdrawal symptoms involve the hydrogen ion (acidity) as the central culprit. The electrical current of injury is initially positive, switching to negative during the healing process.

To initiate an adaptive healing response requires mineral reserves and hormones to mobilize them. Again, the electrical current of injury is initially positive, switching to negative during healing. With the onset of consciousness, the body pools its negative magnetic poles in the peripheral nervous system. Scar tissue and plaque dissolves under a radiant healthy negative magnetic field. They could only have formed because of a lack of oxygen created by an acidic (+) positively charged field. That type of field results from the electrical current of injury. The body heals most effectively in the presence of an alkaline, negative electromagnetic field.

CHAPTER 14

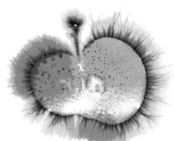

Colloids and the Body Electric

Snowflakes and Colloids

Snowflakes endowed with colloids last much longer than snowflakes without the proper colloids. Like blood or any other fluid, they become congealed when they lack vital colloids. Colloids allow unfrozen fluid to move in chambers within the snowflake. All processes in the body are of an electrical nature and require ion exchange. Salts, acids, and bases that act as electrolytes conductors in our body fluids consist of both anions that carry a negative potential and cations that carry a positive potential. Electrolytes keep blood, body, and digestive fluids in a constant flux of movement.

Mineral colloids, acting as electrolytes, allow extraordinary vitality to ensue. Even though they may appear in only minuscule amounts (parts per billion!), they exert powerful effects. Mineral colloids have extraordinary powers because of (amongst other properties) the microwaves they radiate. Colloids emit a negative, reticular electromagnetic field (alkaline) that catalyzes a change of the electron spin of heavy metals in the body and environment, transforming the metals into inert compounds in the body. The secret of colloids' electrical field and great sensitivity to cosmic forces, along with the bearing of formative forces, resides in the vortices, which the colloids have been spun through. Take our signature beverage, *Electrolyte Lemonade,* which is fresh, raw lemonade, sweetened with raw honey or stevia, with a little living oil and salt. The salt is slowly sun-dried ocean water. These minerals spent eons being tossed about in the ocean before being dried. These electrolyte minerals make the body very elastic and allow old toxins deep within the body to be purged.

Colloids, Galactic Vortices, and Blood

Circulating water spirals in exactly the same patterns as galactic vortices do while creating matter in our universe. In water, colloidal minerals spin in sleeves or layers that move past each other with varying speeds, giving the water a high zeta potential. Zeta potential is the ability of a colloid to retain its charge. The smaller the colloid the greater is its ability to maintain its charge. As larger colloids bounce around, they lose their electrical charge. As the minerals become insoluble, they become less negatively charged. Fresh juice has high zeta potential because the minerals are soluble. As the juice fails to retain its zeta potential, the minerals become sediment.

As a fluid loses its zeta potential, colloids become attracted to each other, making larger colloids. Our whole body is made up of colloids based on circulating electrical attractions. LifeFood colloids impart a charge that energizes the blood cell membrane's protective albumen coating. Charging the cell in this way causes it to be repellent and continuously swept along rather than coagulate. Overall, colloids from Life-Food enhance negative charges of the blood, enhancing its vitality.

Colloidal Nutrients Are Highly Absorbable

Energy is absorbed into the hydrogen bonds of colloids and is released at a lower vibration in the same way that water finds its own level. This is a centripetal motion of energy acting inward and toward its center of rotation, instead of centrifugal, which acts out and away from center. Centripetal energy is the basis for life. Physical and energetic properties of colloids are radically altered by these rotating and electrogravitic forces. By creating a hole or bubble in the ether, colloids manifest a buoyancy or anti-gravity effect. Solubility refers to the ability of an element to remain dissolved in the body fluid and its ability to cross the cell membrane. Both factors are integral components of nutrient assimilation.

The body cell membranes are predominantly made up of hydrogen ions, which tend to be positively charged. Thus, negatively charged nutrients create maximum absorption through cell membranes. This is the process that nutrients go through in the laboratories of our stomach and intestines to make their way into our blood. Nutrients are bound by protein carriers to become miscible with body fluids. The mineral components of these nutrients cross the cell membrane in a chelated form. Electrons flow from a positive pole toward a negative pole. The (counterclockwise) centripetal forces of an alkaline body create a friction grid (implosion) in which tachyons condense into electrons.

Mineral Colloids Are the Condensed Effect of Stars

Colloids of space dust have imprinted resonance. Vibrations are condensed into the mineral colloids of the Earth. These substances are the condensed effects of the stars of our universe. Little do people know that it is living colloids that produce the iron ore that eventually becomes the metal for the engines of the cars we drive. Matter is born from minerals melting and then becoming an ionized gaseous ether (plasma) that electrons and protons are formed from. This observation shows the direct effect of polarization, where negative polarization condenses through its counterclockwise centripetal spin—literally imploding the plasma to form space dust.

Colloids of quartz crystal, when spun in a vortex, change their inertia and tap into forces of the sun and other stars. These forces emit formative resonance that allows minerals to crystallize under certain conditions. Colloids of ordinary quartz crystal, passing through a gravity vortex (caused through stirring), can create millions of aerobic bacteria. Spectrographic analysis shows that the beginnings of silicon dioxide crystals develop minute amounts of various minerals and other elements that are crystallized from the ether.

Colloidal minerals are the enzymogens that, when connected to each other, possess electromagnetic energy. The energy activates their formation into enzymes. Enzymes allow us to biologically transform one element into another, like silicon into calcium. Living cell-like fossils have been found in meteorites from space.

Light is worked into matter through light-bearing elements such as sulfur and phosphorus. Nitrogen guides life to form as the plastics of life (carbon). It is the bridge between oxygen and carbon. Nitrogen, together with hydrogen, sulfur, oxygen, and carbon, forms the protein that composes us. The bearer of internal sensation is nitrogen. It is the nitrogen inside of us that allows us to sense underground water and douse for it with dousing rods, or even without them. Dousing is an ancient trade that determines where to dig for water wells. Of all the elements in the periodic table, silicon and carbon equally exhibit the properties of life. Silicon and carbon are very close to each other on the chart, only one octave apart.

Nutrient colloids subject to electrogravitic forces have their dielectrics stretched. The protons and electrons are stretched away from each other, beneficially widening the electron cloud around atomic nuclei. Naturally occurring electrogravitic phenomena enhance a nutrient's delivery by charging it. The nutrient is made even more soluble as it is reduced in particle size. The greater its surface area becomes the more it is able to maintain its electrical delivery capability.

Charged water that is south-seeking (N-) is highly alkaline forming, transporting alkalizing elements to the most distant places within us. This is significant, seeing that the body is mainly water, because water and oxygen are paramagnetic. The revitalizing and stress-reducing effects on the body from low magnetic field strength (the Earth's magnetic field is currently about 0.5 gauss strong) have been observed clinically and experimentally.

A few hundred years ago, the Earth's magnetic field was as high as 4.0 gauss; only recently has it been waning. Paramagnetic fields are centered in our DNA. DNA repair only occurs in an alkaline medium. Nutrients helping to alkalize body tissue emit subtle, organizing energy fields that help with diverse things, like mineral balance, enzyme function, and DNA replication and transcription.

A base is a substance where hydrogen (H+) ions are few, whereas an acid is a substance where hydrogen ions are concentrated. Acid/alkaline balance is measured by pH (parts of hydrogen), which ranges on a scale from 0 on the acidic end to 14 on the alkaline—with pH 7 being neutral. Thus, body fluids that are above 7 are alkaline, like lymph and blood, while saliva and urine are slightly acidic at 6.8. The lymph is alkaline because it contains a higher concentration of hydroxide (OH-) than hydrogen (H+). Most living matter, excluding the cell nucleus and digestive tract, has an internal pH of 6.8. Blood plasma and extracellular fluid usually have a pH between 7.2–7.3. Some areas of the body, however, could have pathologically developed local areas that were quite acidic or alkaline, even though fluids may have less than reflected this. Buffers are pH-stabilizing mechanisms, minimizing pH fluctuations. Balance is restored when buffers bond with ions, neutralizing them.

Whole brain modes of being, thinking, alkaline-forming LifeFood, coral calcium, microwater, and beneficial negative electromagnetic fields will raise the body's microelectrical potential. As this happens, the electrical potential between a capillary and tissue increases; the selective capacity of cells significantly improves, as do the intracellular and extracellular absorption of nutrients and the excretion of toxins. Only LifeFood can restore this micro-electrical potential. Other therapeutics can augment this function of LifeFood. Oxygen is essential to survival. Although oxygen is stable in the air in an acid environment, is robbed of electrons and its electron orbital shift. A small portion of what we inhale becomes active oxygen due to its unpaired, stabilized proton/electron relationship.

By now you're getting the picture that alkaline nutrient colloids provide many spare electrons for the energy to activate enzymes and promote life itself. As long as we have spare electrons, we have life.

Among the most important nutrients bringing in electrons are essential fatty acids.

Longevity Equals Having Spare Electrons

Essential fatty acids give us an enormous amount of electrons, which help protect cell membranes and produce mineral-mobilizing hormones. The number of spare electrons given to the body by cis-fatty acids, coming from sources like coconut butter, is enormous. If we could be fed all the electrons needed we would live great long lives.

One distinguishing feature of a cancerous cell is the presence of rancid fat in the cytoplasm. In cells of cancer and rheumatic muscle, the membrane of the cell nucleus shows the presence of isolated fat. One could conclude that cancerous masses are condensed and stored material that is without spare electrons and that insulates and blocks the flow of electrons Heating oxidized fats rancidizes it and breeds nu-toxins, like aldehydes.

Essential fatty acids come in the form of LifeFood colloids, including grape seed, hemp, flax, pumpkin, and borage seed oils. They have long-chain fatty acids, which help protect cell membranes from oxidation. They also effectively increase the electric tension on the cell membranes, making them more permeable to oxygen and nutrients. EFAs have many spare electrons in that help sweep toxins along to the liver.

Essential fatty acids protect our cells from oxidation a lot like pre-servatives would. However, most preservatives, like Sodium Benzoate, are respiratory poisons that obstruct the metabolism of fat. Mucous membranes depend upon EFAs for proper function. Excellent blood pressure management and a good ability to handle simple sugars in the diet is often a resolution for fat digestion.

Lymph and lipids are spread over every single blood cell as the life colloids of blood enter the left and right subclavian veins with every squeezing beat of the heart. Lymph and lipid-rich blood enter through the right atrium of the heart, while oxygen-rich blood enters through the left atrium of the heart from the lungs. The difference in blood material creates a differential as the heart contracts, allowing one side to fill as the other empties its contents. This is what governs heart action potentials! If the heart was without essential fatty acids, it would require cytochrome oxidize to help electrons manufacture the important energy-giving ATP.

It Takes Two Poles To Get a Current

Unsaturated fats give us bipolarity just like that of a battery, with a current flowing from the negative pole to the positive. If only one pole is present, the current is unable to flow. Our ability to cope with stress depends upon this "life battery" continuously recharging itself. Unsaturated fats are important nutrients, giving the body the abundance of spare electrons needed to neutralize acids and create energy.

Two electrical poles are needed to create a current of injury or healing; therefore unsaturated fats are integral. When cell membranes are active, they require unsaturated essential fatty acids for body building materials to pass through them. All heat-processed and denatured oils are toxic poisons and should be avoided. That type of fat is unlikely to integrate into lining tissue. It is fat that can be burned, though it is very inefficient and leaves toxic residue from its combustion.

Colloids of essential fatty acids need to be bound to a protein carrier to be miscible with body fluid. The sulfur-bearing amino acid cystine has a positive electrical charge and is an excellent lipotropic protein. Cystine, found in nuts and bee pollen, is capable of emulsifying (bonding water to fat) plant fats. As we will see, though, elements have to have a biotic life force.

As an essential fatty acid from LifeFood binds to its protein carrier, it does a dance around a protein carrier that has an opposite magnetic pole. In contrast, dead fats and proteins would become flatly bound. Live essential fatty acids, as they dance around their protein carrier, fashion a veil of electrons as a cloud of energy. The sun then charges this cloud of electrons.

Electrons Are Our Light Body

Unsaturated cis-fatty acids are rich with electrons and have high cell surface and capillary activities. The closer you go into an atom, the denser it becomes. The farther you go out of the atom the lighter it gets and the less dense its matter is. Electron-rich nutrients move toward the surface. For instance, the capillary activities of lymph and blood flow toward the mucus membranes for elimination through the colon, bladder, or lungs.

The secret of an alkaline body is that it is composed of a large surplus of spare electrons. An electron is lightweight matter. Electrons have a high affinity for oxygen as they crowd to the cell surface, stimulating respiration. We eat about half the food we normally would when we consume *high electric* foods.

Sexuality and fertility functions are related to the important relationship between fats and proteins. Sperm has one thousand times more sulfur-rich protein than any other type of cell. The ovum has very high lecithin and unsaturated fat content!

Living things seemingly move from the dense matter of protons to the light matter of electrons. Human health and vitality is increased as a result of having an abundant supply of electrons.

Organisms larger than a mouse may have seemingly been able to live with the evil pesticide DDT, but if a bird eats a worm laden with DDT its survival is compromised because of its lost electron exchange. More complex animals are more sensitive in their need for electrons. Some organisms carry their battery pack inside, within a central nervous system (astral consciousness), while others rely on an interaction with the energy from the sun for their electrons.

Solar Rays Animate the Electrons of Seeds

In the presence of the suns rays, electrons become stored within the bipolar dance of the fatty acid/protein complex. If you multiply the concentration of solar electrons in this biologically electron-rich complex by a factor of ten, it would be possible to live for 120 years or more. Taking solar electrons into this lipoprotein heightens and maintains our sense of well being. Cheerfulness involves an abundance of electrons as neurons in both hemispheres fire synchronously.

Living tissue stores solar electrons through resonant absorption. Thus, a prerequisite for this absorption and storage is that body and organ tissues possess similar frequencies. Putting cold-pressed coconut butter and Vitamin E on our skin enhances this process. Other kinds of petrochemical lotions, sunscreens, dead oils, or paraffins can cause damage. Protons from cosmic rays and fissioning matter are filtered out through healthy tissue. Yet, excessive pressure placed on a biological system to absorb dysbiotic radiation electrons could cause burn damage or cancers to metastasize.

Cetaceans, like dolphins, are the only well-known life forms that have a higher concentration of solar energy photons than humans. Energy attracts likened energy. This basic law is fulfilled as we consume electrons with solar ray (photon) attractive electromagnetic fields.

Specific Colloidal Mineral Frequency

Colloidal minerals, especially the first thirty of the elementary tables, participate in a wide variety of biological transmutation. Whilst we have health the last thirty minerals, of some ninety that we have in our body, lean over and support the first sixty in their spinning to the right. Otherwise those minerals above sixty on the elementary chart lean in the other direction, influencing things to spin counterclockwise, like uranium. The first thirty-three trace elements emit a wavelength of 2 to 25 micrometers put together in the infrared spectrum. This unique spectrum relieves discomfort and promotes cellular metabolism by helping activate, through resonance, enzymes in helping regulate physiological deficiencies.

The Body Has a Biogenic Energy Field

The body's biogenic field is beyond any ordinary field. Small amounts of this energy have enormous powers. The body's biofield is 100 million times as large as its magnetic field! This biofield of energy produces force at right angles to the body. It appears in the form of spirals, without pushing or pulling like gravity or magnetic fields. This energy has the ability (like a scalar wave) to reorganize the spin of electron clouds. As we know it, this energy can influence enzymes and dissipate structures, without much of a magnetic field. Human hands demonstrate particularly condensed aspects of this biofield that have shown in research to line up hydrogen molecules, aligning the spin of electrons so that one polarity is facing outward to become sweeter and more alkaline. In this situation, blood enjoys greater alkalinity and nutrient/waste surface exchange.

Magnetic fields as much as one hundred times stronger than normal can be detected surrounding human hands with SCQID's (Super Conducting Quantum Interference Devices whose acronym is pronounced "squid"). Even though seemingly small, these barely detectable fields around us affect our biological systems in ways that could only be reproduced with high-intensity electrogravitic fields. This bioenergetic field of negative entropy creates order, even out of seemingly inorganic systems.

Electrons in our food, even vibrations of our thoughts and sounds, stimulate the crystalline structures within us to produce a piezoelectric current. If one has a magnet and runs it up and down a wire, an electrical current is induced in the wire. LifeFood, electric herbs, alkaline-charged microwater, and negative electrical fields all help to oxygenate—and they all supply an abundance of electrons for vital health! Nutrient electrons derived this way have the ability to act as resonance systems for solar energy. Their electro-magneto-gravitic field has the ability to attract photons of sunlight.

Notes

1. Brownian Movement denotes random and chaotic movement of microscopic particles.
2. Radiant Energy is characterized by a specific range of frequency and wavelength of the electromagnetic spectrum in relationship to the related form.
3. Annie Padden Jubb and David Jubb, Ph.D. *LifeFood Recipe Book* (Berkeley, California: North Atlantic Books, 2003).
4. *The Bantam Medical Dictionary, 3rd Revised Edition* (New York: Bantam Books, 2000).
5. Isotonic fluid is a colloid. Mineral elements within the colloid all possess a discreet negative charge, including blood cell membranes. Other plasma proteins have a uniform discreet negative charge on the cell membranes.
6. Pleomorphic organisms are organisms of many changeable forms that have the same origin, such as: colloids, spores, bacteria, mold, fungus, and yeast.
7. Endothelial cells are specialized cells lining all of our passageways. They are delicate cells that are our first line of defense and nourishment.
8. Biological transmutation is the ability in biology to transmutate one element into another alchemically (i.e., organic silica into calcium, potassium into sodium, or manganese into iron).
9. LDLs: Low-Density Lipoproteins. LDLs are an important marker in cardiac infarction risk. Lipids have low solubility in water thus they have to be enveloped in a layer of protein colloids. LDLs carry fat away from the liver HDLs (High-Density Lipoproteins).

10. Reticuloendothelial system cells that are the body's first line of defense, lining passageways within the body that include phagocytic cells (except granulocytic leucocytes). Reticuloendothelial cells as connective tissue fibers refer to those cells lining lymphatic myeloid red pulp of the spleen, etc. Kupffer cells in the endothelial cells that line the sinusoids of the adrenals, liver, pulmonary alveoli of the lungs, etc., are integral for maintaining good albumin levels.

11. Cis-unsaturated fatty acids have a horseshoe shape. Trans-fatty acids have a deranged structure caused because of oxidization. Cis-unsaturated fatty acids are found in all fresh food, and not at all in cooked or denatured food.

12. Isotonic fluid describes fluid that possesses the same osmotic pressure.

13. Somatids (colloids of life) are the very building material of DNA and RNA.

14. Morphogenesis is the development of form and structure of the body and its parts.

15. Homeopathy is a system of medicine based on the theory that "like cures like." The treatments include infinitesimally small doses of medicine that can produce a symptom that is the same as the symptom to be healed in the person. The two symptoms, as waveform patterns, cancel each other out in the same way two equal ripples that meet in a pond annihilate each other.

16. Sacred Geometry is the root of all languages in the universe. It is mathematically sound and reveals a profound order in all things, especially in the codes that create life.

17. Mitosis is a type of cell division in which a single cell produces two genetically identical daughter cells.

18. Mitotic Cell Division is a theory that posits that red blood cells form when one cell goes through a process of division to form two cells. It was first noted in the bone marrow of fasting rats. It is still accepted in many circles, though it clouds the issue of how the *first* red blood cell formed and from where it arose.

19. Hemocytoblast is a formative blood cell.

20. In theory, normoblast cells have a nucleus and are part of the blood-making tissue that gives rise to red blood cells that have no nucleus. This is a fancy theory that we challenge here.

21. Zeta potential is a measurement of energy that comes from the degree of structure in a colloidal system. Fresh orange juice has a zeta potential of about 70 the moment it is juiced and the colloids remain suspended. After a small amount of time a loss of zeta potential occurs and sediment forms.

22. A good read on this theory is *The Aquatic Ape* by Elaine Morgan (Briarcliff Manor, NY: Stein & Day, 1982).

23. DHEA: dehydraepiendesterone. DHEA is a precursor hormone with which other hormones are made from. It is vitally important for mobilization of mineral reserves and managing inflammation.

24. Neoplastic cells are any new or abnormal growth, any benign or malignant tumor.

25. Endothelial system: The single layer of cells that lines the heart, blood vessels, and lymphatic vessels.

26. MHCs: major histocompatibility complex. A series of genes located on chromosome 6 that code for antigens, including the HLA antigens that are important the determination of histocompatibility.

27. Don't forget the trouble that Salomon Rushdie got into during the 1990s when a price of $1,000,000 was put on his head by Moslem extremists in Iran after he published his novel *The Satanic Verses* that superimposed prostitute personalities onto Koran story characters.

28. Half of the procession of the equinoxes (in full 25,920 years) is 13,000 years plus the 900 years we've come since rounding the ellipse corner. Now we are beginning the "Awakening" as we head toward the center of the galaxy.

29. Monatomic colloids are the light elements in the body that provide the energy that cells use to communicate with each other. They give us light to operate and direct our DNA.

30. Tachyons are theoretical particles of unknown density, traveling faster than the speed of light, and about one 12,000th the size of electrons. Tachyons condense through gravitational force to precipitate into electrons.

31. A firme is a unit of measurement that is equivalent to one quadrillionth of a meter, or 10^{-15} meters. Also for reference an angstrom is the width of a hydrogen atom. Hydrogen only has one proton.

32. Planckian frequency is a very tiny, short wave of the kind that interacts with the DNA in our nucleus.

33. Monera are living proteinaceous colloids derived from erythrocytes or digested substance in the villi of the intestines.

34. The body's aura is produced by an electromagnetic gravitic field, the L-field, given off due to the body's ability for superconduction.

35. Adhesion molecules are used by biological systems to hook and anchor. It is the mucus-based material that can bond and connect internal organs to each other when the body is saturated with glue-like foodstuffs.

36. Immune complexes consist of 9 primary proteins involving 27 known sub-proteins, 22 of which are enzymes! These complexes are part of the immune cells ability to neutralize antigens (waste).

37. LifeFood Nutritional Fasting is tissue cleansing, and involves withholding all solid and cooked foods of any kind, while taking in raw juices and blended raw food, including raw blended soup. The diet must be devoid of all starch and flesh for a state of autolysis to occur.

38. NK (Natural Killer) lympyocyte cells are able to kill virus-infected cells as well as certain types of cancer cells.

39. Cytokines are protein molecules that are released by cells when activated by an antigen. They are involved in cell-to-cell communications.

40. Anionic elements are ions, predominantly potassium, calcium, and chlorine, that have spare electrons that are spinning centripetally to the left and are attracted toward the Van Alen belts high in the sky.

41. Larry Dossey, M.D. "Death and hospitals: An inquiry into the body count." In *Alternative Therapies,* Vol. 9(1): Jan/Feb 2003.

42. Diamagnetism is the interface of positive and negative poles.

43. *The Secret Life of Cells*, reprint edition, by Robert S. Stone. (Atglen, PA: Schiffer Publishing, Ltd., 1994). Stone writes of Cleve Baxter's groundbreaking work that reveals how cells respond emotionally to each other and the host body, and how even when separated from the host body cells will respond to the environment and mood of the body.

44. Analogue sculpting is a term coined by Dr. Scout Lee as how the placement of objects in a room can inspire certain emotion or thought, similar in many ways to feng shui, the ancient Chinese art of placement. A book with a meaningful title is placed on a table, or an altar is built in a room to suggest a mood.

    Further, Dr. Lee extends analogue sculpting to the body and its shape and positioning. If you position the body in a certain way you can achieve a certain emotion or mood in the person, "Shape the body and the mind will follow." By observing subtle movement patterns in others, how one opens or closes a door—do you slam it or close it gently?—gives us insight into the deep behavioral structures of the person, how they generally feel and respond to issues in their everyday tasks.

45. Bismuth is a white crystalline metal with a reddish tint. It is a salt employed by the body in many ways, most chiefly because it provides a major protective action of cell membranes, in particular endothelial mucous membranes.

46. A standing wave is a term used to describe the fabric that allows the hologram of life's patterns.

47. Far infrared radiation is the band of electromagnetic radiation that is longer in wavelength than the red of the visible spectrum, it is responsible for the transmission of radiant heat and is used in physiotherapy to warm tissues, reduce pain, and improve circulation.

48. The typical blood pH level in Europe 100 years ago was 7.3. But today most people's blood is about 7.4. Cancer requires a blood

pH of at least 7.56. The proper dextrogyral lactic acid is needed to buffer the alkalinity of the blood. Typically, a person must have an enormous amount of the wrong kind of acids in their tissue for their blood to become alkaline. Blood can also become too acidic. A change in blood pH of just 0.1 can be a matter of life or death.

49. Volutin denotes a basophilic substance, possibly a nucleic acid occurring as granules in algae.

Index

About the Authors

ANNIE PADDEN JUBB

Born in Seattle and raised on Guemes Island in Washington State, Annie moved to New York City in her late teens to study and teach intrinsic properties of health. She has owned and managed raw organic vegan restaurants in San Francisco and Hawaii, and currently in New York City's East Village and Los Angeles. She lives in Los Angeles, providing health readings to clients and overseeing fasts, running corporate workshops, writing and filming, and conducting health research.

DAVID JUBB, Ph.D.

Born and raised on a remote island in Tasmania, Australia, David journeyed to the U.S. to study, receiving his doctorate at New York University. He took two years off to trek the entire length of Africa. An Exercise and Behavior Physiologist, he has devoted the latter part of his career to the anatomy of health. His Health Readings are sought out the world over, as he is renowned for his accuracy in pinpointing the origin of a symptom and how to heal it naturally. David currently maintains a busy private practice in New York City and is always writing and lecturing, both in the U.S. and abroad.

Annie Jubb and Dr. David Jubb have authored nine books together, including *LifeFood Recipe Book: Living on LifeFood, Shamanism: The Path of Formlessness,* and *Cell Rejuvenation,* along with five training manuals for their Whole Brain Functioning adventure-based learning program taught at retreats and lectures throughout the 1980s and '90s. They have had a weekly TV show in Manhattan since 1998. Jubbs LifeFood

Nutritional Fasting Outpatient Clinic, established in 1990, continues to help many thousands each year to safely detoxify, tissue cleanse, and restore good health in the body. The Jubbs maintain private practices in New York City and Los Angeles.

Jubbs LONGEVITY, Inc. is a retail store for all Jubb-recommended products for diet, personal grooming, and home. Enjoy the LifeFood Beverage Bar and gourmet LifeFood Patisserie. When in New York, stop in to pick up everything you need to equip your LifeFood kitchen, purify your tap water for drinking and bathing, and stock up on living whole food vitamins, super foods, and LifeFood treats.

Call for a catalog

Jubbs LONGEVITY, INC.
508 East 12th Street
New York City, NY 10009

Phone: 212.353.5000

www.LifeFood.com & www.jubbslongvevity.com